Alison Roberts has been lu[...]
live in the South of France [...]
recently, but is now back in her home country of
New Zealand. She is also lucky enough to write
for the Mills & Boon Medical line. A primary
school teacher in a former life, she later became
a qualified paramedic. She loves to travel and
dance, drink champagne and spend time with her
daughter and her friends. Alison is the author of
over one hundred books!

Lifelong romance addict **JC Harroway** took a
break from her career as a junior doctor to raise
a family and found her calling as a Mills & Boon
author instead. She now lives in New Zealand and
finds that writing feeds her very real obsession
with happy endings and the endorphin rush they
create. You can follow her at jcharroway.com, and
on Facebook, X and Instagram.

CITY VET, COUNTRY TEMPTATION

ALISON ROBERTS

FORBIDDEN FIJI NIGHTS WITH HER RIVAL

JC HARROWAY

MILLS & BOON

First published in Great Britain 2024
by Mills & Boon, an imprint of HarperCollins*Publishers* Ltd,
1 London Bridge Street, London, SE1 9GF

www.harpercollins.co.uk

HarperCollins*Publishers* Macken House, 39/40 Mayor Street Upper,
Dublin 1, D01 C9W8, Ireland

City Vet, Country Temptation © 2024 Alison Roberts

Forbidden Fiji Nights with Her Rival © 2024 JC Harroway

ISBN: 978-0-263-32174-6

10/24

CITY VET, COUNTRY TEMPTATION

ALISON ROBERTS

MILLS & BOON

For Pauline,
who loves dogs as much as I do.
And for Gracie,
who knows how special she is. xx

CHAPTER ONE

LIFE JUST DIDN'T get any better than this…

Jack Dunlop stood up in his stirrups to get a better view of the mob of sheep flowing down the steep gully towards him. It was late enough in the day for the sun to be sinking behind the spectacular mountain range that bordered this property on the outskirts of Cutler's Creek and that was making it a little more difficult to see everything that was happening despite the cowboy-style hat he was wearing, so he shaded his eyes with his hand.

Then he made a U shape with his middle finger and thumb, wrapped his lips over them and gave a loud whistle.

'That'll do, Bess,' he yelled. 'That'll *do*…'

His dog dropped out of sight amongst the tussock and the sheep slowed down, bunching together to wait, watching the farm dogs warily. Jack waited for his father to appear at the back of the herd, with the other dogs, having rounded up any stragglers amongst the rocky outcrops of the foothills. There was no sign of Dave Dunlop yet, but Jack was more than happy to take a moment to enjoy the scenery and he relaxed into his saddle again and turned to look towards the old family homestead—a solid stone, two-storied house that had been built well over a hundred years ago. The dwelling might be on the other side of the main road that divided the property, but both the house and ancient shearing shed looked as much a part of this New Zealand landscape as the mountains on this wilder side of the road.

He reached down to pat his horse's neck and loosened the reins to let him stretch his head down to find a few blades of grass.

'How lucky are we, Custard?' he mused out loud. 'To live in a place like this and spend an hour or two out here after work to unwind with the girls.'

The 'girls' were a small mob of around a hundred and fifty sheep. It had started as no more than a way of keeping the grass down in the hard-to-reach places of the gullies in the foothills, but Jack had become interested in breeding these sheep with naturally coloured fleeces in all shades of black and brown and it was now an enjoyable hobby that he could share with his dad. They were rounding them up to take them into the yards, down on the flat land between the shearing shed and the house. Jack had brought the portable ultrasound scanner home so they could find out how many lambs each ewe was carrying and plan their supplementary feeding for the next few weeks.

There was no guarantee they'd have the time to get the scanning done as well as the mustering, though. As the only veterinary surgeons in this rural community, one of them always needed to be backup even if they weren't formally on call because another out-of-hours vet could be based miles away or busy on another job. Besides, knowing that nobody around here would call them out during the night unless it was a real emergency, they would both want to do whatever they could to help an animal in trouble on their patch.

If his father didn't appear anytime soon, they might even run out of time to get them down the road and into the yards, anyway. Jack made a clicking sound with his tongue and Custard's head came up instantly. Bess the dog stood up, waiting for instructions as she saw Jack move in her direction.

'Stand there,' Jack commanded.

This wasn't going to take long. He could see the other dogs appearing from the gully now, driving a couple of wayward sheep. Then he saw his father's horse, a black mare called Mary.

And it was in that moment that he could feel the solid foundation of his life starting to tilt.

Because the saddle was twisted sideways and his father was nowhere to be seen...

The sheep scattered as Jack raced up the hill as fast as Custard could manage. He hurled himself off the horse as he got through the entrance to the gully and saw the shape of his father lying flat on his back on the rocky ground.

'Oh, my God, Dad...are you okay?' He crouched beside the older man. 'What happened?'

Dave Dunlop had his eyes shut. 'Not sure,' he said. 'I think Mary slipped on a rock. We both went down. She... I think she might have stood on my back... I can't feel my legs and my hands feel all weird and tingly...'

A chill ran down Jack's spine. 'Don't *move*,' he said. 'I'm going to call for help.'

They were not only lucky enough to have a hospital in Cutler's Creek but one of the local doctors, Isaac Cameron, was qualified as a specialist trauma surgeon. He was also one of Jack's best mates. So was Ben, the senior paramedic in their ambulance station.

'I'm on my way,' Zac told Jack as soon as he got the call. 'I'll get Ben on the road with the ambulance as well, but I have a feeling we're going to need a chopper. I'll get them on standby. Don't let your Dave move a muscle and support his head so he can't move his neck.'

'Onto it,' Jack said.

He ended the call and then knelt on the hard ground. He put his hands on either side of his father's head, spreading his fingers to provide the best support he could.

'I'm sorry, son…'

Dave sounded as though he was in severe pain and Jack's heart broke.

'Don't be sorry,' he said, his voice rough. 'It's going to be okay. We've got through worse than this in the past, haven't we?'

'You're not wrong there, lad,' Dave said quietly. 'And yeah… We'll get through this as well.'

As dawn broke the following morning, however, Jack found himself fighting to retain that optimism.

It wasn't simply that he was exhausted physically after a sleepless night.

He'd been part of a huge emergency response that had involved a good chunk of the close-knit community he'd grown up in. Bruce, the chief local policeman, had arrived along with Zac and Ben with the ambulance and coordinated everyone coming along the road who had stopped to offer assistance.

A neighbouring farmer had taken the horses away to take their saddles and bridles off and shut them safely into a paddock beside the Dunlops' house. A nurse on her way home from the hospital took the dogs back to their own kennels and promised to stay overnight to care for them. The sheep were in the far corner of their paddock, tightly bunched in a frightened huddle.

Jack had become part of the medics' determination to give his father the best of care, helping to immobilise him on a back board with his body, head and neck carefully secured with straps, cervical collar and tape. IV access was obtained and pain relief given, along with fluids and other drugs that could control complications that a spinal cord injury could cause, such as falling blood pressure and shock. They kept him warm and comfortable and reassured, monitoring his vital signs as they waited for a rescue helicopter to arrive. Even secured as well as he was, no one wanted to risk making a high spinal injury worse by carrying him down the steep, slippery slope to a ground surface that was flat enough for a helicopter to land, so it became a winch operation.

A small, visibly shocked crowd gathered on the road to watch the rescue of a man who'd devoted his life to caring for their livestock and pets and it was in that moment that Jack was reminded of his mother's funeral, where these same people had gathered to watch him stand beside his father, only five years old and bewildered by the turn that life had taken. The effect of that memory was to ramp up the fear for his father. And for himself, although he couldn't let himself go anywhere near the horror of losing his only parent—the man who'd raised him alone and created a bond that made him the absolute rock in Jack's life.

Jack had run on adrenaline as he made arrangements to have a vet in the closest town cover Cutler's Creek for any emergencies in the next few days and travelled with his father in the helicopter to the nearest specialist spinal injuries team and the intensive care his father might well need. Several hours later, the results of the scans were enough for the doctors to be cautiously hopeful that Dave might have escaped a life-changing injury and paralysis, but he needed urgent surgery and would be having a halo neck brace fitted, attached to his skull with metal pins, that would protect his neck as it healed.

It was still an emotional rollercoaster for Jack as he paced the floor of a relatives' room, waiting to be allowed into Recovery to see his father after the apparently successful surgery.

He was, in fact, close to tears as he watched the sun coming up.

Life could change in an instant, couldn't it?

There he'd been, thinking that life didn't get any better than it was for him, but the shock of an accident that could have been catastrophic had left him realising how wrong he'd been.

What would he have in his life if he'd lost the person who was his only family? The most important person in the world to him?

He'd have a job he loved.

A community that was like an extended family.

He'd have his beloved dogs and his horse and a home he wanted to live in for the rest of his life.

He'd have his friends, like Zac and Ben. Even a couple of ex-girlfriends who had been able to cope with only being in his life—and his bed—for a limited time.

Okay…that was a lot. More than many people had in their lives, for sure.

But it wasn't really enough, was it?

Because Jack had had a glimpse of being in his home with only his dogs for company and he'd seen the truth.

And he didn't like it.

It *was* a great life, but it wasn't quite what he'd dreamed of.

It would, in fact, be what he'd most feared when he'd been that frightened five-year-old who'd just lost his mother.

It would be…unbearably lonely…

Andrea Chamberlain was not having the best day.

'I'm so very sorry, Mrs Parker.'

The elderly woman had her hand pressed to her mouth and tears streaming down her cheeks. A small dog was lying on the high table between them and was now watching its owner with the kind of deep concern spaniels were so good at displaying. Andrea stroked the silky black head and gave him a reassuring ear rub.

'We can keep him comfortable for a little while yet,' she told her client. 'But there's nothing more we can do. The MRI scan has shown us just how far the cancer has spread now. I'm so sorry,' she said again, swallowing back her own tears. 'I know this is the last news you wanted to hear.'

And she knew exactly how hard this was going to be. Janice Parker lived alone with a dog she absolutely adored.

Just how Andrea felt about her own fur baby, Pingu.

Losing a beloved pet who had been such an important part of your life was always devastating. She'd seen—and totally empathised with—the fear in Janice's eyes when she'd rushed her fifteen-year-old Cavalier King Charles spaniel, Toby, into the clinic a couple of weeks ago, having felt a hard lump in his abdomen. Toby had had a lumpectomy, which he recovered from quickly, but when the aggressive nature of the cancer had been identified, a scan was done to see if a chemotherapy course might be an option.

It wasn't.

And it was only a matter of time before the kindest thing to do would be to make sure this little dog didn't have to suffer. Thankfully, this appointment was the last one for Andrea this afternoon and she could take as much time as she needed to make a plan of how they could both help Toby get the best quality of life and the most happiness out of whatever time he had left.

Andrea stayed in the consulting room for a few minutes after Mrs Parker had carried Toby back to the reception area. She pretended to be tidying shelves that contained all sorts of supplies and medications, but she was actually trying to get her head together so that she could face her colleagues without revealing the level of difficulty she'd had coping with that last appointment.

Being too emotionally involved with a case could count against her in her bid to become one of the permanent partners of this practice—a goal she'd been working towards ever since she'd been lucky enough to score a locum position in what was the place she had dreamed of working ever since she'd decided to become a vet.

A position that she'd been in for nearly two years now, but while the invitation to become a partner had been hinted at, it had not yet been formally extended. Perhaps it was because she was feeling so bad about Mrs Parker and Toby that her longed-for goal seemed further away than ever. She certainly didn't feel inclined to stay late, as usual, to catch up on paperwork, chase lab results or go over details for the surgeries on her list in the morning. She could do all that later tonight.

What she needed to do right now was to go and give her little dog a cuddle and then take him home. Pingu had a large, comfortable crate at the back of the hospital wing, where he snoozed between short walks or visits whenever Andrea could take a few minutes' break in her working hours. Everybody here loved Pingu and helped look after him and that was another reason why she was so keen to make this job permanent.

When that happened, her life would be perfect...

Andrea opened the door of the consulting room to find the practice manager, Ginny, right in front of her.

'Andi...are you free for a few minutes?'

'I can be. What's up?'

'Warren wants to see you in his office.'

Warren was her boss. Everybody's boss, here. He had set up his own small veterinary practice at least forty years ago not long after he'd graduated from vet school and he'd built it into the most prestigious and successful small animal practice in the city of Auckland.

Ginny's eyes were wide. 'It sounds like he wants to talk to you about something important.'

She knew how much Andrea wanted to join the practice. She also knew that Warren had the casting vote for the employment—or firing—of every staff member. She leaned closer to Andrea and lowered her voice to a whisper.

'Maybe this is it. The *offer*...'

Andrea's heart skipped a beat. Maybe it was.

She tucked a wayward strand of hair behind her ear before she knocked on Warren's office door.

'Come in... Ah... Andi. Just the person I wanted to have a chat to. Do sit down...'

Warren's smile suggested that he was delighted to see her, in fact. As if he had some really good news he wanted to share, even. Andrea was smiling back as she sat down on the comfortable leather chair to one side of the antique desk that was Warren's pride and joy.

'You've become a real asset to this practice,' Warren said. 'I'm hearing that you're getting more and more referrals for orthopaedic surgery, which is hardly surprising given how well you've done in your postgraduate training. It's the perfect area for you to specialise in, going forward, and it would be a good investment for us to facilitate any further training you want to do. Or set you up to get involved in some research.'

Andrea's breath caught in her chest. Funding specialist training or research projects was not something that would be done for a locum who could move on at any time.

'Top of the agenda for the next partners' meeting is drawing up a partnership agreement for you, Andrea.' Warren was still smiling.

Yes...!

But Warren's smile faded slightly. 'I do need you to do me a small favour in the meantime,' he added.

'Of course,' Andrea said. 'What is it?'

But Warren gave her a thoughtful stare before he spoke again.

'How old are you, Andrea?'

'Thirty-four.'

He nodded slowly. 'I was quite a few years younger

than you when I started this practice, but it's been my life's work and it's something I'm very proud of. It almost didn't happen, though...'

'Oh...?'

Warren shrugged. 'I couldn't afford it, even though it was much cheaper in those days to set up a clinic of your own. I was lucky enough to be offered a loan. My closest friend all through university—a man called Dave Dunlop—was setting up his own practice in Cutler's Creek. He mortgaged his house to do it and he wanted to help me have the same opportunity, so he lent me the money.'

'That's an amazing thing for someone to do. He must have been a very good friend.'

'He still is,' Warren said. 'I paid the money back, with interest, long ago, of course, but I suddenly find I've got the chance to help him as much as he helped me back then.'

Andrea had no idea why this was relevant to her potential partnership. She was also slightly distracted by the mention of a place called Cutler's Creek. Why was that name familiar?

'He was lucky to survive a fall from his horse a week or so ago. Even luckier that his cervical injury hasn't resulted in paralysis. He's been allowed to go home to recuperate, but he's got a halo brace screwed into his skull and hardware attaching it to some kind of rigid chest harness, so he won't be working for at least three months. He contacted me to ask if I knew of someone who could come and help his son run the practice while he's out of action. Mixed practice. Rural and small-town stuff.'

Did he want Andrea to find a potential locum?

'Where is Cutler's Creek exactly?' she asked.

'South Island. Central Otago. About an hour or so out of Queenstown. Gorgeous place, from what I've heard. Mountains, lakes, rich gold-mining history...'

But Andrea wasn't listening now. She didn't want to hear about Central Otago. About a place she'd avoided even thinking about since she'd been five years old. Because she hadn't wanted to go anywhere near that nightmare again.

'So I told him I had the perfect person.' Warren's voice broke through Andrea's defence system. 'Someone who can turn her hand to anything and do it well. So well that we're intending to offer her a partnership.'

'Me...?' Andrea's voice came out as a horrified gasp. 'Oh, no... I'm sorry, but that's not possible.'

'Oh?' Warren sounded surprised. 'Why not?'

'Because I live *here*. I have a dog. An apartment full of pot plants.' Okay...maybe that wasn't a very good reason. 'Clients who are depending on me,' she added quickly. 'Like Mrs Parker. I had to tell her that Toby's condition is terminal today.'

The quirk of Warren's eyebrows made her feel as if she was stooping to using emotional blackmail by bringing Mrs Parker and her old dog into this equation.

'None of that needs to be a problem,' he said smoothly.

Unless you choose to make it one, his look suggested.

'I will look after Mrs Parker and Toby personally,' he assured her. 'Dave said he's more than happy for you to bring your dog with you and I'm sure your concierge can look after your apartment and water your plants. It won't cost you anything for accommodation, either. Dave's got a big old house that's been in the family for generations, but there's also a shearer's cottage if you prefer to be independent. He's also happy to reimburse you for any travel costs, like the ferry crossing and fuel.'

Andrea could feel her head turning slowly from side to side.

No…no, no, no…

Warren's gaze was steady. He wasn't smiling now.

'I owe this man,' he said quietly. 'If it hadn't been for his faith in me and his generosity, this practice wouldn't exist. Your job wouldn't exist.'

Oh, help… Was she supposed to feel grateful to this unknown old friend of Warren's? Grateful enough to go somewhere she'd promised herself she'd never have to go again?

'I'd go myself, but I can't abandon a large practice that I'm responsible for.' Warren raised his hands, palms outwards in a gesture of defeat. 'I'm also the chairman of the committee that's running an international veterinarian symposium happening in less than eight weeks and we've still got a huge amount to organise.'

He was holding Andrea's gaze. 'I would be very grateful if you could do this for me. Very grateful indeed.'

And there it was. The offer of a partnership had been made but only informally. It could easily be rescinded if Andrea demonstrated that she wasn't prepared to be a team player and put the best interests of the practice—and the stranger who'd made it possible that it existed in the first place—over any personal reservations.

She wanted this job.

It would be the final feather in her cap of total success.

To fail in her goal to be a partner would mean that all her hard work and focus and personal sacrifice since she'd been old enough to recognise that perfectionism and success got you noticed—and valued—had been for nothing.

The position as a partner would be the icing on the cake that, so far, consisted of her gorgeous penthouse apartment, the stunning Porsche 911 sports car that she'd managed to score in her favourite shade of Guards Red and, of course, the most adorable fur baby in the world.

All good things. But the real status, the real respect and acknowledgement that other people thought she was something special, would come from becoming a partner.

Andrea didn't just want this job.

She *had* to have it... She couldn't allow herself to fail.

She managed to summon a smile, even.

'Fine,' she said. 'How soon would you like me to go?'

'It'll be at least a two-day drive, even with that flash car of yours.' Warren was smiling back at her. 'I suggest you get sorted tonight and hit the road first thing in the morning.'

CHAPTER TWO

IT WAS STILL THERE...

Small, white wooden crosses were often hammered into the ground on the side of New Zealand roads to mark where a tragic car accident had occurred. If one had been placed recently, it often had some flowers attached to it, or even a photograph.

This one, however, had been here for almost thirty years and Andrea Chamberlain was probably the only person who was still aware of its significance. She hadn't planned on stopping to look at it—quite the opposite, in fact. But she'd recognised this patch of the road, probably because it had haunted her dreams ever since the accident. The slope of this hill where it had been carved through the rocky ground. The bridge over the small, fast-running stream at the bottom before the curve that took the road up the other side of this gully.

There was a rest area on the other side of the bridge—a shingled space big enough for several cars to park, trees shading a picnic table and a track that led down the river to provide access for fishing or an opportunity for a tired driver to stretch their legs. It hadn't been just for Pingu's sake that Andi pulled off the road to stop for a few minutes. She might have prepared herself for the flash of memory that she knew she wouldn't be able to avoid as she came down the hill towards the bridge, but it was so much sharper than she had anticipated it had stolen her breath away.

She needed to try and centre herself and put these memories somewhere they couldn't make these next few weeks unbearable for her.

Andi left the roof down on her car as she clipped a lead to Pingu's harness and walked down to the river. Carefully. On their last stop for a snack and fuel, she had changed into the smart, casual outfit she wanted to be wearing when she met her new, temporary boss. White jeans, a dark blue fitted denim shirt and stylish but comfortable shoes in her favourite slingback style. White, of course, to match her jeans, but the kitten heels made them a bit slippery on the rough stone pathway.

It was a very warm spring afternoon and the air was fragrant. There were butterflies and bees drifting amongst the pink flowers of brier roses and she could smell wild thyme being crushed beneath her feet.

'This is where I grew up,' she told Pingu. 'Well, not here exactly because we're nearly at Cutler's Creek. But I lived just outside Queenstown with my mum and dad and it was…'

…perfect, that's what it had been. Not that Pingu was interested. He was dipping his white, fluffy feet into the icy cold water of a mountain stream. A curly poodle cross, he was all white apart from where he was black around his eyes, had black ears and a big patch on his back like a black saddle blanket. He'd looked like a penguin when Andi had seen his photo as a newborn puppy, so it had been easy to find a name for him.

When he'd had a paddle and a drink and Andi had recovered her courage, she led him across the bridge. The cross that some long-forgotten family friend had put up was almost hidden amongst a colourful patch of orange and yellow Californian poppies and that was when the tears prickled at Andi's eyes.

Her mother had loved these cheerful, little wildflowers and she could remember picking bunches of them. Not here, of course. She wasn't quite sure how she could be so certain they hadn't been growing here back then. Maybe the idea that her mother had somehow made it happen was too irresistible. A touch from an angel? An apology to that small girl who'd been trapped in the car seat that had kept her perfectly safe in the mangled wreckage of the car. Waiting and waiting for someone to come and help.

For someone to make her parents wake up because they were so fast asleep in the front seats that they couldn't hear her crying for them.

Andi stooped to pick one of the bright flowers. She tucked the stalk behind her ear. It was then she became aware of a new sound nearby. One that was just as familiar as the sound of cicadas even though she hadn't heard it since her childhood—the slightly anxious sounds a flock of sheep made when they were being kept moving but weren't quite sure where they were going. The muffled barks of more than one dog were close enough to be a warning that these sheep were coming around the corner on the other side of the bridge.

'Come on, Pingu. We'd better get out of the way.'

But Andi was a moment too late in tightening her hand around the end of his leash. The little black-and-white dog had also heard the barking and the calls of the sheep and he pulled the leash from her hand and he was off, running to find out what was going on and barking as loudly as he could.

'*Pingu... No...*'

He couldn't hear her. Or he didn't want to hear her. Pingu was over the bridge now and the excitement of being near this crowd of huge creatures with his own sort of woolly coats was too much. To the disgust of a farm dog who was doing its best to control the mob from the front and the farmer on a horse on the other side, Pingu was dashing this way and that, barking non-stop and… bouncing to make himself look bigger and more ferocious. Watching the sheep scattering in all directions— into the rest area, down the track towards the river, over the bridge towards Andi and past the horse to go back the way they'd come—Pingu's attempt at being a sheepdog was a resounding failure.

The man on the big palomino horse was shouting and whistling.

'Get away, Jazz…'

'Come over, Bess… *Stand*…'

'Speak up, Meg…'

Black, tan and white farm dogs were barking and racing back and forth as they responded to the curt instructions to try and undo the chaos Pingu was creating. Andi had her arms out wide and was making noise of her own to try and stop the sheep taking off in a panicked run past her and down the road where there could be oncoming traffic. She was also yelling at Pingu.

'*Come* here, Pingu…' She was using her strictest voice. 'Right *now*…'

Not that she could see if she was being obeyed. Her

small dog had vanished in the forest of sheep legs, but she could hear his higher pitched, excited barking despite the noise of the other dogs and the background calling of anxious sheep. Andi tried to lean sideways to spot where Pingu was, but as she came off the bridge and into the entrance of the rest area, she slipped on the rocks and found herself sitting on a patch of the road that more than one sheep had been using as a toilet.

'Oh…*yuck*…' Andi scrambled to her feet, wiping her hands on her jeans. One of the farmer's dogs gave her a very disparaging sideways look as it ran past with its head down, and when Andi lurched forward and discovered that one of her heels had snapped clean off her shoe, the only thing that stopped her bursting into tears was the appearance of a contrite-looking small dog with a filthy lead trailing behind him. His white paws—his whole legs, in fact—now looked as though he'd been wading through a patch of mud, but Andi knew that it wasn't mud that was making them look this disgusting.

And, okay…maybe there was something else that was making her fight those tears. The farmer on his horse had stopped beside her and he was looking down at her with a rather similar expression to the one she'd just seen on his very well-trained dog. A dog who, with its mates, had already succeeded in calming the sheep and had them corralled in the rest area, surrounding her low-slung sports car.

The man looked like he'd ridden out of a Western blockbuster movie. He was in black from head to toe. Boots, jeans, a tee shirt and a cowboy hat. He had a darkly shadowed jaw and…

…and he was nothing like any man that Andi would ever consider suitable to date but…

…but she had to concede that he *was* absolutely drop-dead gorgeous—with that kind of rough diamond, bad boy…yeah…*cowboy* vibe.

He was also more than annoyed. Andi fully expected him to tell her exactly what he thought of her for not having control over her dog and putting his livestock at risk, so she was totally disarmed when he did speak.

'Did you hurt yourself?' he asked calmly. 'When you fell over?'

Oh, my…those tears were even closer now, but for a very different reason. This modern-day cowboy actually sounded as if he cared and, given the fragile emotional space she was being forced into by being here, it touched something that went far deeper than Andi was comfortable with.

So she glared at him.

'No,' she said. 'I'm fine.'

She had to be one of the most beautiful women Jack Dunlop had ever seen. A famous model, perhaps? Or a celebrity he didn't recognise? The Lakes District with its mountains, lovely lakes and picturesque towns was a tourist mecca, so he wouldn't be at all surprised if she was here for a photoshoot or to make a movie.

Long waves of sun-kissed blonde hair flowed over her shoulders onto a fitted denim shirt that had the sleeves rolled up and a button or three undone at the front. Not that he could see much thanks to the fluffball of a dog she now had clutched in her arms.

Had she flown in on a private jet so that she could

bring her designer dog slash emotional support companion with her? And then hired the glitziest car on offer from a high-end rental service? They might have something to say about her transporting a now very dirty little dog who probably smelt like the back end of a sheep. His A-list owner wasn't going to find a dog grooming salon anywhere nearby, either. Jack's lips twitched.

'You might want to throw him in the river.'

The suggestion came out in what was supposed to be a thoughtful drawl, but the horrified look on her face made him hear his words from her point of view.

Oops...

'Just to get him clean,' he added. 'You probably don't want him messing up the inside of that flash car of yours.' He turned his head to the car that was a red island in the middle of his flock of sheep. 'What is it? A Ferrari? Lamborghini?'

'A Porsche,' she muttered, her gaze sliding away from his.

At least she had the grace to look embarrassed. She was the archetypical fish out of water, wasn't she? A city princess who had found herself in the wrong place at the wrong time. Those stains from wiping her hands on her white jeans as she'd scrambled to her feet after that fall would probably never come out completely and he'd seen the way she'd been walking like a drunk pirate with a wooden leg thanks to breaking the heel off her shoe.

He couldn't deny how attractive she was but, thankfully, that was the biggest red flag ever. He'd given in to that kind of attraction before—fallen hard enough to end up marrying the kind of woman who favoured white jeans and high heels—and that might be well in the past now, but he wasn't about to forget what a disaster it had been.

There was no point being angry with her, either, and telling her what a liability she was on a country road and that she'd put his valuable, pedigree sheep in danger. Jack pulled the brim of his hat down in case he failed to prevent the smile that was trying to form. What with the state of her clothes and her dog, she was probably being punished quite enough. She might well have also broken a finger-nail or two, in that brush with the tarmac.

'Where are you headed?' he asked. 'Queenstown? Wa-naka? Arrowtown?'

'Cutler's Creek.'

Jack blinked. He was about to ask her why on earth she was heading to his hometown when she began to turn away.

'I'm sorry Pingu chased your sheep,' she said. 'I'll get out of your way if you can move them enough for me to get to my car.'

Pingu?

Good grief...

'He's black and white.' The stranger didn't bother turn-ing back to him. 'It's the name of a penguin.'

Jack bit his lip. He hadn't realised he'd spoken aloud. He let his breath out in a sigh, wondering if he should apologise, but then he let out a piercing whistle instead.

'Let's go, girls...' he called. 'Party's over...'

The old, two-storied stone farmhouse was easy enough to find, a kilometre or two down the road from the rest area, and if Andi had been in any doubt that she'd found the right address, it was dispelled as a man opened the door with his head encased in a metal band that was locked with straight rods onto some kind of device he was wearing under his shirt.

'Mr Dunlop?'

He had to be horribly uncomfortable walking around with all that ironmongery holding his head still, but he had the warmest smile Andi had seen since...

...oh, *my*...

Was it because she'd just visited where it had happened and because she'd been thinking about him that made this man remind her so clearly of her own father? Made her remember even more poignantly how much she had adored him and how much she had missed him ever since he'd been ripped out of her life?

Andi could almost hear the echo of a terrified child's voice in the back of her head.

Wake up, Daddy... Please wake up...

The reaction was gone in a heartbeat as the man spoke again.

'And you are?'

'Andrea Chamberlain. I work for Warren. You asked him to find you a locum for your vet clinic?'

He was looking astonished. '*You're* our locum?'

'Yes. Did you not know I would be arriving today?'

'We knew the locum was arriving, but we were expecting a bloke. Andy. Short for *Andrew*, not Andrea.'

'Is it a problem?'

There was relief to be found in the thought that this visit might be a lot shorter than she'd expected. She could turn round and get out of this patch of the world with its minefield of memories and ridiculously good-looking farmers with their perfectly behaved dogs who would never chase a sheep unless they'd been told to. She could drive the length of the country back to Auckland having demonstrated that she was a team player and deserved that partnership. It was probably fair enough that Warren's old mate didn't want a female locum. What if they had a two-tonne bull that needed surgery or something?

But…

'No, no…of course not. It's a bonus, that's what it is…' That smile was back again. 'I'm so sorry—that was incredibly rude of me. Please come in. You must be worn out after all that driving.' He had to tilt his whole upper body to look over her shoulder. 'Weren't you going to bring your dog with you?'

'He's still in the car. He's a bit damp.' Andi stopped short of telling the entire embarrassing truth. 'He had a bit of a swim when we stopped at the rest area down the road. You might not want him in your house until he's dried off, Mr Dunlop.'

'Call me Dave. We don't stand on ceremony around here. And go and get your wee dog. We've had way worse than a bit of damp tramped through this house over the years, let me tell you…'

He was going to tell her. This rural vet, whom she guessed to be the same age as her father would have been by now, was clearly a born raconteur and she could imagine him leaning on a farm gate with his clients just having a yarn or simply telling stories after he'd finished doing whatever he'd gone there to do as part of his job.

He took her—and Pingu—through the house to a wonderful old country kitchen that had an ancient cast-iron stove built into a brick chimney and a lovely old hutch dresser that was crammed with rose-patterned crockery.

'Cup of tea?' he offered. 'No…what about a glass of wine? Our neighbours have a small vineyard and they make a very good pinot noir.'

'A cup of tea would be fabulous,' Andi told him. 'But I'll make it. I'm guessing you're supposed to be resting as much as possible.'

'Thanks, love… I could do with sitting down for a bit.' He touched one of the metal rods attached to the halo ring. 'This thing is heavier than it looks.' Something changed in the older man's face and Andi got a glimpse of just how hard this man's life had unexpectedly become. How much pain he was in and the effort he was making to be so cheerful and welcoming.

Her heart went out to Dave. She liked him. A lot.

'How do you take your tea?' she asked. 'Or…would *you* prefer a glass of wine?'

The twinkle was back in his eyes. 'I'm only allowed a small glass,' he said. 'But…let's celebrate your arrival. Just don't tell Jack when he gets home.'

'Jack?'

'My son. Your new colleague for the next month or two.'

'I won't tell,' Andi promised. 'And I'm looking forward to meeting him.'

Her words were quite genuine. If he was anything like his dad, this blip in her life plan could well be way more enjoyable than she had anticipated.

No *way*…

What the hell was *that* red car—that was probably worth more than his entire flock of sheep—doing parked outside his home?

Jack Dunlop kicked his heavy boots off on the front veranda and marched into the house. Bess, his favourite dog,
slunk along just behind him. She knew her master was
in a very uncharacteristically bad mood all of a sudden.

He had been looking forward to going straight to the
kitchen to get a cold beer from the fridge after the hard
work he'd just put into what had become a much more difficult task than it should have been. The sheep had been
thoroughly put on edge by the disruption to being moved
to another paddock and seemed to be expecting another
fright from a fluffy soft toy come-to-life apology for a
dog. They'd all been tired by the time it was done and the
dogs needed to be fed and put in their runs and the horse
brushed down and given a biscuit of hay.

Jack was hot, grimy, knew he didn't smell very good
at all and he was hungry.

He was on the edge of being distinctly hangry, in fact,
and the sound of laughter—feminine laughter—coming
from the terrace at the back of the house was the last thing
he wanted to hear.

Was the movie star, model, princess-in disguise still in
her filthy white jeans with a broken shoe?

No. She was wearing faded blue jeans now and had
what looked like a designer brand of trainers on her feet.
She must have brushed her hair since he'd last seen her
because it flowed like silk over her shoulders onto a close-
fitting white tee shirt that did nothing to hide her curves.
Jack hastily averted his gaze, but it wasn't fast enough to
stop that curl of sensation deep in his gut. The one that
reminded him of just how attractive this woman was and
how that reminded him that women like this were…

…dangerous, that's what they were.

Curled up beside her, on the soft cushion of the wicker couch, was the small dog who'd seen them coming well before the people did. It was wagging his silly curl of a tail and looked ready to launch itself at Bess in an invitation to play.

Bess froze.

So did Jack.

Bess growled.

Jack didn't. But only because the blonde woman had looked up and he had the satisfaction that his presence alone was enough to wipe the smile from her face. It almost looked as if most of the blood had drained away from it as well.

Was she *scared* of him?

That thought was disturbing, to say the least. Jack Dunlop had never done anything that could scare a woman. Quite the opposite. He took his hat off and flipped it sideways to land on the large, low coffee table. A brief glance at Bess stopped another growl and his dog went to curl up on her bed beside a pizza oven that was built into this paved terrace shaded by a pergola that was almost invisible beneath the spring foliage of a couple of exuberant grapevines.

Bess was glaring at the visitors.

So was Jack. He couldn't help himself.

His father didn't notice. Probably because he couldn't turn his head and he was too comfortable, propped up with so many cushions around him that he didn't want to turn his body. That empty wine glass might well have something to do with how relaxed he was.

'Jack…' His father sounded happier than he had since

before the accident. 'You're not going to believe this, but this is Andi. Andi, meet Jack—my son.'

'Andy?' Jack couldn't summon even a hint of a smile. 'Our...locum...?'

'That's the one.' Dave was having no trouble smiling. 'Short for Andrea, not Andrew. Bit of a surprise, eh?'

'That's one word for it.' Jack's tone was as dry as his throat that was still coated with dust. He desperately needed a moment to himself. He had to think fast and find his way out of the situation he'd walked into. A totally ludicrous, unacceptable situation. This was going to be the shortest locum position ever. Because it wasn't even going to start.

'Excuse me...' he muttered. 'I need to wash my hands and find a beer.'

'Find me another drop of wine while you're there, would you?' Dave gestured towards the empty glass in front of him. 'Andi only poured me a mouthful and that was after checking every milligram of medication I'm on. Oh, and turn the oven on. Maureen's left us a steak-and-mushroom pie and some baked spuds for dinner that just need heating up.'

Sluicing his face and hands thoroughly with cold water in the kitchen sink gave Jack enough time to come up with a plan. He took the bottle of red wine back outside with him, along with his lager. There was no reason not to be polite about this.

'Top up?' he offered.

'Yes, please,' his father said.

'I was actually talking to Andi.'

'Thanks,' Andi said. 'Gorgeous wine, but I won't have any more.'

'I'll have hers, too.' Dave grinned. 'It's not as though I'm going to be driving anywhere.'

Jack poured him just another mouthful or two. His gaze slipped sideways as he did so, to find two black eyes like buttons staring at him from the couch. The odd tail wasn't wagging this time, however. Penguin dog didn't like him.

The feeling's mutual, buddy...

He was careful that he didn't say that aloud. At least the dog's legs were considerably cleaner than the last time he'd seen him. He flicked a glance at their human visitor.

'River?' he asked succinctly.

She nodded. 'It worked really well. I held on to him and dangled him up to his belly in a fast bit of the current. I think he liked it.'

Jack grunted. He took a long swallow of his icy cold lager as he sank into a single chair opposite his father. He eyed the poster child of designer dogs again. 'What *is* he, exactly?'

'A schnoodle.'

'Sorry?' His lips twitched. 'Or should I say "bless you"?'

Andi wasn't amused. 'He's a first-generation cross between a schnauzer and a poodle. A small one. Both parents were the miniature varieties of their breeds. Yours is a heading dog, yes? Mostly border collie?'

Jack paused with his bottle in mid-air, that embryonic smile evaporating. 'Yeah... Bess is a heading dog. How did you know she isn't a huntaway?'

'She's smaller and wasn't barking like the other dogs. And there's an intensity about heading dogs that's different, isn't there?'

She must have sensed his surprise. 'I might be in an

inner-city practice now,' she added, 'but I did my share of farm work in my training and when I was moving around the North Island before I joined your dad's friend in Auckland and managed to get back to my inner-city comfort zone.'

'Warren,' Dave put in. 'I told you about him. Best mates we were. He said he'll miss her, but he's happy for Andi to stay here as long as we need the extra help.'

'But we don't need the extra help.' The words didn't come out quite the way Jack had planned when he'd been washing his face in the kitchen, but that description of a city being a 'comfort zone' had been a bit of a trigger, hadn't it? 'I realised today how well I've been managing on my own since you've been out of action.' He eyed Andi over the rim of his bottle to see how she was taking the rejection. 'I'm sorry you've had such a long trip, but you're welcome to stay the night before you head back.'

'Hang on a minute...' Dave said. 'You don't get to make a decision like this on your own, son. I might be out of action, but we're still partners. I've got as much say in this as you have and I think Andi should stay. You might think you don't need the extra help, Jack, but we both know there's too much work for one vet here. And how do you think you're going to manage a major trauma or surgery single-handed?'

The two men stared at each other and the silence quickly became charged. Maybe that was why Andi got up from the couch.

'Excuse me,' she said. 'I'm just going to find the bath-room.'

'Second door on the left as you're heading for the front door,' Jack told her crisply.

Her dog gave him a dirty look as he followed Andi.

So did his father.

'Did you have to sound like you expect her to keep walking right out of the house?' he growled.

'Best if she does,' Jack responded. 'She's a city vet, Dad. She'd be totally useless here. I don't have the time or inclination to be mollycoddling a princess who probably spends her time looking after overweight designer dogs or...or guinea pigs or something. I don't *want* her here.'

'Well, I do.' Dave's tone was adamant. 'I suspect she's a lot more skilled than you're giving her credit for. Warren certainly seems to think highly of her. He's planning to offer her a full partnership in his practice and that's highly sought after, I can tell you...'

'You didn't see her this afternoon. She and that dog just about had my entire mob scattered along the main highway or trying to head downriver. Stress like that could bring on early lambing.'

'Takes two to tango,' Dave snapped. 'You were in charge of those sheep. I like her,' he added firmly. 'I want her to stay and...and that's that.'

Andi wasn't intentionally eavesdropping.

She hadn't deliberately let the lace of her shoe come undone or stooped to retie it before she was halfway across the stone slabs of this rustic country kitchen, but there it was.

She'd heard every word that was being said about her out on the terrace.

When she straightened up again, she needed to take a deep breath and find the courage to not do something 'princessy'—like burst into tears or walk straight out of this house and drive off into the sunset.

Of course she wasn't going to do something like that.

She'd been far too young when she'd learned not to let her heart rule her head. That you could only get what you wanted by staying in control. Or, at least, get closer to what you wanted because nothing was ever going to be able to give her what she wanted most in life—that self-esteem that could only come from being loved unconditionally as a child. From being part of a family.

That her being a female vet might be a problem should have been welcome. She'd be able to escape the challenge of facing old memories of when her world had been ripped apart that she knew were going to test her. Oddly, the cowboy vet making it crystal clear that he totally agreed with her had, rather dramatically, completely changed her mind.

It wasn't simply because her head was reminding her that a promotion to partner in her dream clinic might be threatened if she left Warren's old mate in the lurch.

Or that his old mate's son thought she wasn't suitable because she was a woman and needed to be shown how wrong he was.

No…what had really done it was that he thought she'd be *useless* in the career she was passionate about.

And he'd actually said aloud that he didn't want her here.

He couldn't have found a more effective trigger to provoke an emotional reaction that went so deep.

A potent mix of fear and grief and…shame?

Yes. The shame of realising that you weren't good enough, or special enough, to be wanted…

She could hear, and feel, echoes of her grandmother's reaction to having to come and collect her after the death of her parents and take her away to Auckland to bring her up. Another overheard snippet that still hadn't lost its power despite the passing of so many years.

I suppose I'll have to...but another child is the last thing I want to have in my life...

But the cowboy's father wanted her.

He liked her. He knew she had to be good at her job or Warren wouldn't be offering her a partnership.

He wanted her to stay. He was facing his own challenges right now, but he'd gone out of his way to make her feel welcome.

Wanted...

She loved him for that.

And damn it. If Dave Dunlop wanted her to stay, then Andi *was* going to stay.

Jack was welcome to find another locum that he found more acceptable, but Andi was going to stay until he did—for Dave's sake. Who knew...maybe that would be enough time to prove to Jack that she wasn't useless. That there *were* reasons that people could very much want to have her around.

She really wanted to prove that.

It wasn't just to have the satisfaction of watching Jack Dunlop eating his words.

Maybe she needed to prove it to herself as well.

CHAPTER THREE

IT WAS WARM enough to eat outside, under the grapevines, at a wooden table with bench-style seats on either side. Jack and Dave sat opposite Andi. Pingu was tucked under the bench by Andi's feet and Bess the heading dog was sound asleep by the pizza oven.

The halo brace made it a lot more difficult for Dave to eat.

'Ignore me,' he told Andi. 'I've regressed to being a small child and having my food cut up for me. I tend to drop it on the floor sometimes, too.'

'You're doing fine.' Jack was cutting his father's food into small, bite-sized pieces. 'They said it would take time to get used to being in the brace.'

'How long do you have to wear it?' Andi asked.

'Twelve weeks or so, if things heal well.'

'It must be hard to sleep in.'

'I'm sleeping in a recliner chair at the moment. With plenty of pillows to prop me up. I'm told I'll get used to it and be able to sleep in bed again soon but, in the mean-time, poor old Jack's become a carer on top of every-thing else he's got on his plate. I have to say, though, that I wouldn't want anyone else doing it. I'm very grateful I've got him.'

'And I'm very grateful you didn't manage to kill yourself,' Jack growled. 'So we're even.'

Andi caught the look that passed between the two men. She could feel how close they were and it gave her an odd ache deep in her chest. How wonderful would it be to have an unbreakable family bond like that?

She envied them. So much.

Jack's tone lightened. 'How 'bout less talking and more eating?'

'The pie's delicious,' Andi said, as encouragement.

'Maureen's a good cook.' Dave was stabbing at his plate without looking down. 'She started out more than forty years ago as my receptionist in the clinic and then trained as a vet nurse, but she's been a kind of house-keeper for us ever since we lost Jack's mum when he was only a wee lad.'

'Oh… I'm sorry to hear that.' Andi risked a glance at Jack. He might not like her or want her here, but they had something big in common, didn't they? He'd been lucky enough to still have one parent, though, and the love between them was clearly as solid as the mountain ranges in this part of the country.

He didn't see the glance. He was reaching out to spear some food Dave had been chasing around the plate and then put the handle of the fork back into his father's hand before he took a bite of his own meal.

'So…' he said, eyeing Andi. 'What made you want to become a vet?'

'I found I liked animals more than most people.'

Dave snorted. The corner of Jack's mouth lifted in a half smile and it felt as if a little bit of ice had been broken.

'Favourite animal?'

'I do quite like guinea pigs.'

She could feel the moment Jack realised she had over-heard what he'd said earlier. She looked up to find a pair of dark eyes watching her steadily and the crinkles at their corners made his expression apologetic. It also made him look very like his father.

Another small chunk of ice melted away. She smiled just enough to let him know she wasn't necessarily going to hold his derogatory comments about her against him. She might even offer him a 'get out of jail free' card.

'Being a country vet is not something I'm likely to be either good at or enjoy,' she admitted. 'I love the small animal practice I'm in. If you find someone more suitable as a locum, I won't be offended, but I'm happy to stay and fill the gap until you do.'

Jack and his father shared a glance. The way Dave raised his eyebrows was the kind of look a parent gave a child whose behaviour had been particularly disappoint-ing. Andi knew that look all too well. Her very existence, let alone her behaviour, had been a constant disappoint-ment to her grandmother. She felt a twinge of compas-sion for Jack.

'Dogs,' she said into the awkward silence. 'They're my favourite. And horses, though I don't get to see too many of them these days.'

'Do you ride?'

'I do. I did, anyway. Haven't had my own horse since I left school.'

'You could keep my girl exercised while you're here, if you fancy a ride,' Dave said. 'She's a nice wee bay. Mary.'

'Because she's a mare?'

Andi and Dave shared a smile. They got each other.

'She behaves herself most of the time,' Dave added. 'She's not too mareish.'

'She's a station hack,' Jack muttered. 'She'd be no good for doing dressage in a paddock. Likes a good run up the hills and a bit of jumping.'

The warmth of any compassion Andi had been experiencing wore off instantly. With a mouthful of food that excused her having to speak, Andi simply made a sound that could have been acknowledgement that she wouldn't be able to manage a farm hack. She wasn't about to tell Jack that she'd competed, and done well, in national three-day equestrian events, so she wasn't as useless as he thought she was.

She wouldn't pass up an opportunity to make him look apologetic again, mind you.

'Wouldn't mind trying a run up the hills while I'm here,' she said, casually, having swallowed her mouthful. 'Sounds fun.'

'You could take her out with Custard,' Dave suggested. 'Show her the boundaries of the farm or go along the river trail.'

'Custard?' Andi used the same disbelieving tone that Jack had when he'd echoed Pingu's name after hearing it for the first time. She could feel her smile stretching across her face. 'Is that the name of your palomino?'

'He came with the name of Custard Pie,' Jack muttered. 'I didn't choose it.'

'It's a great name,' Andi murmured. 'Very yellow.'

This time, when Jack lifted his gaze, she was the one watching him. She was still smiling and, after a beat, Jack smiled back. A proper smile, as if he was genuinely amused. Giving her credit for standing up for herself?

Touché...

It was the first time she'd seen this man really smile and...it had been worth waiting for.

He was good looking enough when he was broody and bad tempered, but when that smile lit up his face, he looked like an advertisement for a new series of reality television—the one where the bachelor got to take his pick from a bevy of beautiful women. Or the matchmaking one where the farmer went looking for a wife.

Whatever...

The smile was certainly doing something very strange to Andi's body—creating a sensation that made her think again of the ice that had been around them at the start of this meal. It wasn't bits breaking now, however. It was more like it was melting fast enough to trickle right down to her bones.

She might not like this man much and he was definitely not her type at all. She could see why a great many women would find him irresistibly attractive, but that laid-back, slightly scruffy, roguish charm wasn't for her. Even if it had been, this man had actually said—*aloud*—that he didn't want her.

She could—and would—put a stop to that melting sensation. This level of physical response to a man was not only unwise, it was dangerous. There would inevitably be an emotional component to that response and that only made any conflict between the heart and the head harder to control. This unwanted awareness of Jack Dunlop was only there because she was tired. And because she'd been thrown into the deep end of an emotional pool that she hadn't wanted to even dip her toes into. But Andi was well practised in staying away from the kind of emotion that could interfere with a focus on what was important.

Like success. Respect. Appreciation.

She could cope with this.

She'd coped with far worse in the past, after all.

Jack could see that his father was tiring by the time he'd finished eating.

'Let's get your pin care done and let you get some sleep,' he suggested.

Dave nodded. 'Then you can show Andi where the spare bedroom is. Or the cottage. You could give her a tour of the clinic, too.'

Jack didn't say anything as he collected the plates. While he would have preferred not to be sleeping under the same roof as this visitor, there wasn't much point opening up the old shearer's cottage for just a night or two. With a bit of luck, after sleeping on it, his father would realise how unsuitable Andrea Chamberlain was as their locum and they could find someone else fast.

It wasn't simply because she was an impossibly attractive city princess who wore white jeans and heeled shoes and looked like she had her hair professionally streaked and styled on a regular basis.

Or even that it was way too much of a reminder of the disaster his marriage had been after he'd fallen for exactly this type of woman. That year from hell might be ancient history now, but man, the effects could linger, couldn't they?

No…there might be some very personal factors in his distaste for this situation, but they were outweighed by professional reasons. This was a mixed country practice and there was a lot of heavy, difficult—sometimes dangerous—livestock to wrangle. Andi had admitted herself it wasn't the kind of work she was interested in or would even like.

Jack didn't want to send his father's friend's potential new partner back to Auckland with an injury that could be life changing. He was looking after her, that's what this was about. The faster he found a replacement, the better. For both of them.

Having satisfied himself that he would be doing the right thing by sending Andi packing as soon as possible, he showed her where the spare bedroom was and then went to help his father clean the pins on his halo to protect his skin from infection, made sure he'd taken his medication and was comfortably set up in his reclining chair to watch a bit of television and then, hopefully, get a better night's sleep tonight.

Andi went outside to give her dog a walk before bringing her bag in from her car.

Twenty minutes later, when he heard the sound of tyres crunching on the shingle of the Dunlop's long driveway, Jack actually thought Andi might be doing a runner. He walked to the front door, expecting to see the taillights of the Porsche disappearing into the distance and wondering how he would break the news to his father that the woman he'd taken such an instant liking to was too rude to even say goodbye face to face.

What he found, instead, was a farm ute parked in front of the clinic building and someone he knew very well lifting a large, shaggy dog from the tray of the vehicle.

'Terry…' he called. 'What's going on, mate?'

'It's Jed. He's done himself a mischief. Think he might

have broken his leg.' He put the dog down on the ground and it stood, looking miserable, with a hind leg held up.

'Oh, *no...*' Jack was striding towards him. 'And the trials are at the end of next week.'

It was then that he saw he wasn't the only person approaching these out-of-hours clients. With Pingu at her heels, Andi was only a couple of metres away.

'Sheepdog trials?' she queried.

'Regional championships,' Jack said. 'Jed here is the favourite to take out the huntaway zigzag and straight hill runs. Up against my Meg, who's actually pregnant to Jed. Oh, *man...*' He gave Terry a sympathetic grimace. 'Let's get him inside and see how bad it is. What happened?'

'He was running downhill, jumped a wire fence and landed funny. Gave a bit of a howl. He can walk on three legs, but he hasn't put any weight at all on that back leg since. Come on, mate.' Terry scooped the large dog back into his arms. 'I'll give you a lift.'

'Have you got X-ray equipment here?' Andi and Pingu were following them as Jack punched in a code and led Terry into a deserted reception area. 'Preferably digital?'

'Yes. And a well-equipped operating theatre. Dad and I cope with all the routine surgery and we can call in a specialist surgeon occasionally, but if it's something complicated or urgent, we stabilise them and send them through to a larger facility in Queenstown or Dunedin.'

'I'm registered with the Australasian Veterinary College as a specialist orthopaedic surgeon if that's any help.'

Jack paused with his hand on the door to one of the consulting rooms, turning to stare at Andi. For some obscure reason, learning that she was more qualified than himself was...a little embarrassing?

Because he'd been so quick to assume that she'd be so useless as a country vet that he'd actually said it out loud—and she'd heard him?

Or was it because he would prefer her to be the one who was impressed? With *him*? Not that he was about to give the question of why that might be any headspace right now.

'You're a specialist? In veterinary orthopaedic surgery?'

Andi stared right back. 'Yes. Isn't that what I just said?'

Terry was staring at Jack as well.

'Um…this is Andi,' Jack told his friend. 'She's…ah… come down from Auckland to help while Dad's out of action.'

Terry was staring at Andi now. 'Guess that's a stroke of luck, then. She can have a look at Jed, yeah?'

'Yeah.' Andi nodded. 'Bring him in and put him on the table.' She took off the cardigan she'd put on to go walking outside and dropped it into the corner of the room. 'Bed, Pingu,' she ordered calmly.

The little dog instantly lay down on the cardigan and put his nose on his paws to watch Andi from afar.

Jed was panting and clearly in pain.

'We'll need to give him some sedation and pain relief,' Andi said. 'We can't examine him properly or take X-rays if he's not relaxed.'

Terry had his hand on his dog's back. 'Do whatever you need to, Doc.' The big, burly farmer's voice had a wobble in it. 'This one's special…'

Jack drew up the drugs needed to get Jed comfortable, sliding a gaze or two sideways to watch Andi gather what she needed from the shelves. She was watching Terry, who still had his hand on his dog.

'He's a good-looking dog,' she said. 'Good splash of Beardie in there, yes?'

'Yeah…along with some border collie and Labrador. Bit of Rottweiler back a few generations as well, I reckon, with that black-and-tan colouring, but you wouldn't know it. Jed here's a gentle giant.'

'I can tell. He's lovely.' Andi had a tourniquet, razor and cannula in a kidney dish, ready to insert an IV cannula in the dog's front leg, but she didn't do it immediately. Instead, she offered the back of her hand for the dog to sniff and then put it gently on the scruffy head and scratched behind his ear.

'Hey, Jed…' she said. 'You're a good boy, aren't you? We're going to look after you, okay?'

Jack could see the way the dog was looking up at Andi with that complete trust that never failed to melt his heart. He could see Terry looking at Andi with a rather similar expression, except his trust was mixed with the desperate hope that this injury wasn't as bad as he feared. As if Andi was a magic fairy who could wave her wand and make everything better.

Jack watched the deft way Andi slid the needle into a vein in Jed's front leg and secured the cannula. With the dog drowsy and relaxed within minutes, she started a thorough examination of Jed's back, hips and legs.

She obviously knew what she was doing and her calm competence was…well, Jack had to admit it was sexy on a whole different level to anything physical.

'Nothing's obviously broken,' she told Terry. 'But we'll confirm that with some X-rays in a minute. Given the way he injured himself, I'm thinking it's probably a CCL tear. That's the cranial cruciate ligament in the knee joint—it prevents the tibia moving forward on the femur. Canine equivalent of the ACL in humans.'

Terry blew out a breath. 'Tore mine playing rugby when I was in high school. Hurt like hell.'

'Given that he's not putting any weight at all on the leg, rather than just limping, it's more likely to be a full rupture than a partial tear.' Andi positioned her hand on the top of Jed's back leg and took hold of the lower part of his leg with her other hand. She moved it, carefully, backwards and forwards.

'See that?'

'What is it?'

Jack answered for Andi. 'In a normal, stable joint, we shouldn't be able to move the tibia like that. That's telling us that there's some significant cruciate ligament damage. I think Andi's right in thinking it's a complete rupture.'

Andi reached out to stroke Jed's ears again. 'Good boy,' she said. 'I'm nearly done.'

This time she took hold of the dog's foot with one hand while she had the index finger of her other hand on the patella. She flexed the hock and nodded at the movement she could see. Jack was also nodding. Andi knew what she was doing.

The X-rays confirmed there were no fractures to add to the diagnosis.

'It may not be a complete rupture,' Andi told Terry, 'and some partial tears can be treated successfully with medical management like rest, physio, laser therapy and joint supplements but, in my opinion, this injury is severe enough for me to say that surgery is the best option.'

'I'd say it's the only option,' Jack added, 'if you want him to get back to having a joint that's fully functional. The CCL is under more stress in dogs than the ACL in people because dogs always have their knees bent.'

Terry was rubbing his forehead with his fingers. He swore under his breath. 'Jed lives for working the sheep,' he said. 'I've got to get him right. He's only four, so he's got a lot of good years ahead of him.' He looked up. 'How long will it take?'

'The surgery?'

'No…to get him back to being able to work.'

'Best-case scenario, he should be back to near normal in three months or so,' Andi said. 'No more than six months for complete recovery in most cases.'

'You won't want to be competing with him until we give him the all-clear,' Jack added.

'A brace can help accelerate healing time,' Andi said. 'Keeping things secure after surgery can help prevent any setbacks. Have you got any in stock, Jack?'

'No. But we can measure the size needed and order it. He won't be able to use it for a few days, anyway. Until the swelling's gone down after the surgery.' He caught Andi's gaze. 'Are you thinking TPLO surgery?'

She nodded. 'Especially for a big dog like Jed.' She turned to Terry. 'I won't go into all the details unless you want me to. Basically, it means removing all the damaged bits of ligament and cartilage and then we change the shape of the top of the tibia, reposition it and hold it in place with a plate and screws.'

'Will he have to stay here?'

'Might be a good idea for tonight,' Jack said. 'So we can keep him comfortable and make sure he's nil-by-mouth.

That is, if Andi's happy to do the surgery first thing in the morning? Otherwise I'll need to see if they can fit you in for emergency surgery in town.'

Andi caught his gaze the instant he turned and there was a lightning-fast silent exchange between them.

Sorry about before... I know you're not useless. I could really use your help here.

Forget it. This isn't about you. It's about a dog who needs help.

'Of course I'm happy to do it,' she said aloud. 'I'll have a wander round the theatre tonight and make sure we've got everything we'll need. All going well, he should be able to go home tomorrow evening.'

'He'll only be able to have a few very short walks a day, on a lead, for the next couple of weeks,' Jack put in. 'And nothing high impact, like running or jumping for eight to twelve weeks, but we can start some physio and the brace will help.'

Terry swallowed visibly. He looked from Jack to Andi and back again. Then he glanced at the little black-and-white dog in the corner of the room, who was still gazing adoringly at Andi, and Jack could see him relax a fraction.

She knew, didn't she? How important a dog could be?

'If it's any comfort,' Andi said, 'I get patients sent to me from all over Auckland for exactly this surgery. Mostly dogs, but some cats, too. Even an alpaca last year. Prize stud who got kicked by an unappreciative female. He was back to work twelve weeks or so later, completely recovered.'

She was smiling at Terry. 'Leave him with us,' she said quietly. 'We'll take the very best care of him, I promise.'

Jack caught his breath. The way she was looking at

Terry and that tone in her voice. How could you not trust
this woman? If the skills she'd displayed in her examination of Jed were an indication of her surgical ability,
then Terry had hit the nail on the head earlier, hadn't he?

It *was* a stroke of luck that Andrea Chamberlain had
turned up in Cutler's Creek.

He was watching her like a hawk.

He was watching Jed, too, of course because it was
Jack who had administered the anaesthetic and was now
monitoring the dog's breathing and other vital signs as
he assisted Andi with the surgery, but it felt as if his eyes
never left her hands.

Was he holding his breath, perhaps, as he waited to find
out whether he'd done the right thing last night in asking
her to do this surgery?

That eye contact that hadn't been long enough to be
significant but had still seemed to convey both an apology for the things she'd overheard Jack saying about her
and a surprisingly humble request for assistance.

Andi had gone to sleep last night thinking that his ability to admit he was wrong, along with a willingness to ask
for help on behalf of someone else, was a trait that a lot
of men didn't possess and it made him...more likeable?

Intriguing, even?

Not that she was thinking about him at all now that
this surgery had begun. She couldn't blame Jack for his
intense scrutiny, either. Andi wasn't just responsible for
the future career of the champion sheepdog on the table in
front of her. She was operating on the beloved workmate
of one of his friends. The father of a litter of pups one of
his own dogs was due to give birth to in a few weeks.

It was just as well she was in her comfort zone here. This was a procedure she was more than comfortable with and she'd spent her whole life being a perfectionist, so it wasn't really surprising that Jack was making the occasional impressed sound as he watched her work, removing all the damaged tissue and then making a circular cut at the top of the tibia and rotating the bone fragment.

'Nice,' he murmured. 'It's a clever idea, isn't it? Making the ligament redundant by removing that slope and making the joint stable.'

'It's very satisfying when you've got a procedure that's academically quite simple but very effective when it's done well.' Andi glanced up as she reached for the stainless-steel bone plate that would be screwed into place to hold the bone fragment in position. 'Sometimes, when I'm shaving a bit of bone to make it fit perfectly, I remember that orthopaedic surgeons used to be thought of as carpenters.'

It sounded like Jack was smiling beneath his mask. 'And neurosurgeons were the electricians.'

'And cardiology was just a bit of plumbing.'

The shared amusement changed the atmosphere and Andi no longer felt like she was being assessed. It felt more like she was being appreciated.

Admired, even?

Whatever it was, she liked it.

A lot.

Focused again, she finished the surgery and closed the wound on Jed's leg and Jack reversed the anaesthetic and made sure the dog had plenty of pain relief on board before carrying him to a comfortable crate in the recovery area.

'I'll give Terry a call and let him know what a good job

you did,' he said. He'd broken the top string of his mask to let it dangle around his neck, so Andi got the full wattage of that amazing smile. 'Thanks, Andi.'

'Thank *you*,' she responded. 'I couldn't have done it on my own.'

Jack had, in fact, showed exactly how competent he was in this environment. Andi suspected he would do a good job in whatever challenge was put in front of him. They'd both been assessing each other, which was perfectly normal for people who'd never worked together before.

Whether she got the chance to see the whole range of his skills was another matter. He'd been happy that she was here and could do this surgery, but it wasn't farm work, was it?

Finding a more 'useful' locum was probably next on Jack's to-do list for today.

CHAPTER FOUR

A WEEK HAD gone by and no mention had been made of any new locum coming to take her place.

Andi had been introduced to Maureen on her first day on the job, just after she'd finished the surgery on Jed the huntaway. Maureen was in her sixties and was more than happy to act as either or both a receptionist and vet nurse for Cutler's Creek Animal Hospital—with duties of cleaning and cooking thrown in on a regular basis.

'Don't you do any of the tidy up in Theatre, love,' had been Maureen's initial greeting. 'I'm a dab hand at using the sterilizer and dealing with contaminated linen. Just give me a list of anything that needs reordering, too.'

The older woman had the warmest smile and loved nothing more than to stop for a chat.

'Jed's doing well,' she told Andi later that morning. 'And I've just met your dog, who's quite happy in his crate. I don't think I've ever seen anything as cute. He reminds me of those sheep. You know? Those Swiss ones with the black faces.'

Andi had to shake her head. 'I don't know them.'

'Have a look online and you'll see what I mean. Any-hoo…don't you worry about your pup. I'll look after him if you get called out for a farm job.'

But Andi hadn't been called out for any farm work in the last week.

Going out with Jack in his double-cab ute with all his gear in the covered back tray on the afternoon of her second day was the closest she'd got to any large animal work and that was only to see a pet goat who needed his hooves trimmed.

George the goat lived in the township of Cutler's Creek and driving through was the first look Andi had at this small, rural township that couldn't be less like her hometown in New Zealand's largest city.

'This is the main drag,' Jack told her as they headed past a rugby field and then a modern building that was the shared headquarters of the local emergency services of ambulance and fire response. 'Actually, it's the only drag. We'll go to the other end so you can see everything. It won't take long.'

He drove with his elbow resting in the gap provided by having his window rolled right down, but he had his fingers on the steering wheel so he could use his other hand to point out the local attractions.

'We're lucky enough to have a good supermarket. Saves driving too far to get the groceries. The cafés are good, too, if you're missing a decent, big-city flat white.'

The war memorial that was a feature of every small town in New Zealand gave Andi an unexpected pang of nostalgia. A pull into the past that was almost as powerful as the view of the mountains that were the stunning backdrop to the town.

She had avoided coming back to this part of the country for her whole life. She'd even avoided reading articles or letting her gaze linger on any photographs of Central

Otago because it was preferable not to trigger the automatic link to traumatic memories.

But...she hadn't just turned her back on what was the most beautiful part of this country, had she? She'd dismissed the place she'd been born. A landscape that was part of her heritage. The place where her childhood had been idyllic.

Where the world and everybody in it could be trusted.

Where she'd been safe to love because she'd been loved so much.

The reminder that the trauma of having that destroyed meant that she could never trust the world or anyone in it to the same extent was painfully poignant but, for the first time, Andi was grateful that she'd been forced to come here. Perhaps this would bring closure so that she could go back home to Auckland and not be haunted by the part of her life she hadn't ever dared tap into.

'That's our community hall.' Jack's cheerful voice broke the silence. 'Been to a few good parties there.'

'I'm sure you have.' Andi grinned. 'Bit of line dancing?'

Jack tugged on the rim of his cowboy hat. 'Yes, ma'am.' He slid her a sideways glance. 'Don't knock it till you've tried it. What do you do in Auckland for fun? Yoga? Tai Chi? Boot camps with a personal trainer?'

'All of the above.' Andi nodded. She didn't mind the teasing. It was a reminder that, while she had a significant connection to this part of the world, it wasn't her home and that made it safer to be here, because it gave her a place to escape back to eventually. 'What's that big building coming up? The local hospital?'

'Yep. Cutler's Creek Community Hospital. My friend

Zac's one of the doctors there. It's small, with only about ten beds, but there's an emergency department and a theatre for minor procedures. I'm trying to persuade him to get an MRI machine installed so I can use it for an extension to the animal hospital. Right...here's the road we're after. Have you trimmed a goat's feet before?'

'Can't say I have.'

'I don't think it'll be much of a challenge for you.' Jack threw her a wry smile this time. 'Not when I've seen you shaving a few millimetres off the head of a tibia.'

The look he was giving her made Andi remember the way she'd felt during that surgery. How pleasant it had been to feel that admiration. The twist in the smile that he was giving her didn't make it different enough from that first one to prevent a flash of that melting sensation, either, and the combination made it quite difficult to break that eye contact.

It was probably just as well Jack broke it as he shook his head. 'Lucky it's dry today. We'll stop at the hardware store on the way home and get you a pair of gumboots. Those trainers of yours might be good for boot camp, but they won't stay looking that clean for long around here.'

Andi opened her mouth to suggest that the purchase wasn't necessary if she was only going to be here for such a short time, but then she stopped herself saying anything.

Something had shifted between herself and Jack when she'd told him about her postgraduate qualifications and it had been strengthened as they'd worked together on Jed's surgery. It might be only temporary and professional, but they were feeling their way into some kind of relationship here, and if this was a game of chess, the next move was Jack's, not hers.

Passing a school playground with a surprising number of children running around made her break the silence, however.

'That's a lot of kids. I thought Cutler's Creek was a small town.'

'School bus brings them in from all over the district.' Jack had raised an eyebrow. 'You don't like kids?'

'Love them,' Andi said. 'As long as they're someone else's.'

'Not keen on any of your own, then?'

How could she have ever wanted to have children of her own? To bring utterly vulnerable babies into a world that could be upturned and leave them alone and unwanted. Unloved and so very desperately unhappy...

But Andi kept her tone light. 'Absolutely not. Unless they're of the fur variety. You?'

'Me? Yeah... I want about six of them—the two-legged kind. I was an only child and that house of ours needs more of a crowd.'

Wow...if being a cowboy or playboy or just a plain bad boy hadn't been enough to make Jack Dunlop an unwise choice in men, the fact that he wanted a houseful of kids put him on a different planet as far as comfort zones went.

Not that it was a problem, mind you. It was none of her business. Andi even managed an impressed expression.

'Who's the lucky woman, then?'

'What?'

'The one you've chosen to be the mother of all those kids?'

'Oh...' Jack was pulling the ute to the side of the road. George the goat could be seen on his chain, grazing the long grass along the fence line. 'Haven't found her yet.'

He killed the engine. 'Some things you need to be a bit picky about, you know?'

'I couldn't agree more,' Andi said. 'And life partners and kids are definitely on the top of that list.' She was staring through the windscreen. 'George has large horns, doesn't he?'

Jack laughed. 'Maybe this will be a challenge for you, after all.'

Jack had always intended holding the goat's horns to keep Andi safe while she trimmed the goat's hooves with a pair of secateurs. He hadn't been at all surprised that she'd made a good job of the task, either, even though it was at the opposite end of the skill spectrum from what he witnessed in Theatre that first morning.

That surgery on Jed had changed his opinion of her dramatically. With that mane of blonde hair stuffed inside a cap and her body hidden beneath baggy scrubs, it had even been easy to forget that she looked more like a model than a vet, and watching the absolute focus and precision of the way she handled the surgical instruments to get exactly the result she wanted advertised not just years of study and practice but a level of skill that many surgeons never achieved.

Jack had been seriously impressed.

Jed had gone home with Terry the same day, and by the time he came back to be fitted for the firm, elastic brace that would support the joint towards the end of the week, both dog and master were looking much happier.

Jack was much happier, too.

He hadn't stopped being aware of what an attractive woman Andi was, mind you, he was just able to overlay the response his body was determined to have by re-membering that this was a professional arrangement. It wasn't as if it could ever be anything else, anyway. City girls were out-of-bounds. Another disaster waiting to hap-pen. Jack had been bitten hard enough to be forever shy of them. As a colleague, however, he was quite happy to have Andi around.

It was far more useful than he'd thought to have a city vet in residence. It left him free to head out to do the farm work without worrying about emergencies coming into the hospital or routine work like check-ups and vaccina-tions, laboratory tests and repeat prescriptions piling up. Maureen had fallen in love with Pingu and was clearly delighted to assist Andi with clinics and minor surgery and his father was enjoying her company out of work hours. They had really hit it off, for some reason, and Dave Dunlop was, in fact, looking happier than he had since his accident. The distraction of having someone who hadn't heard all his stories before and was genuinely en-joying them, along with the excuse for a glass or two of wine before dinner as he told them, was giving his father something to look forward to every day and that could only help make his recovery less of an ordeal.

That was enough all by itself to justify keeping the status quo, so one day was leading into the next and Jack hadn't got around to trying to find a locum with experi-ence of working in a mixed practice. Andi hadn't asked how the search was going. She had said that she'd be happy to bridge the gap, so maybe she wasn't in any hurry to leave?

And maybe Jack wasn't in any particular hurry for her to leave, either.

Bess had even stopped growling at Pingu. She was just ignoring him now and Pingu was sensible enough to be keeping a respectful distance.

He didn't move when he saw Jack and Bess coming through the French doors onto the terrace this evening, however. Perhaps he felt safe because he was sandwiched on the couch between his father and Andi, who was holding up her phone high enough that he could see the screen when he couldn't bend his neck.

'Maureen told me about them the other day,' Andi was saying. 'But I only had a look today. She's right. They're super cute, aren't they?'

'What are?'

Andi looked up at the sound of Jack's voice.

'Valais Blacknose sheep,' she told him. 'Known as the cutest sheep in the world. Look...' She handed him her phone. 'Look at those adorable black faces and ears. They've even got black socks and knee patches.'

Jack grunted and handed the phone back. 'There are more important traits than looking cute.'

'I think I want one,' Andi said. 'Maureen was right. They're the ovine equivalent of Pingu.' She smiled at Jack. 'You could get some. Your dad told me that you've got designer-coloured sheep. These guys would fit right in.'

'My mob is designed to produce coloured wool of the highest quality,' Jack said. 'Not just to look like fluffy toys.' His sniff was offended. 'We've put years into not just breeding for colour but for the fineness of a low micron, staple length and crimp and lustre. Our wool is snapped up by craftspeople for spinning, weaving and knitting. Besides, some of my lambs are just as cute as those ones. You'll see for yourself in a few weeks' time.'

Good grief…had he really just said that he expected Andi to still be here at lambing time?

Pretty much admitting that he wasn't even going to try and find a different locum?

Was that why Andi was giving him that odd look?

Apparently not…

'My mother used to spin,' she said quietly. 'And knit. I remember helping her wind the wool into balls.'

'Past tense?' Dave enquired gently.

Andi simply nodded. 'I lost both my parents in a car crash,' she said. 'I was probably about the same age as you were, Jack, when you lost your mum.'

Jack blinked. He would have said he had nothing in common with Andi other than their profession. That they couldn't be further apart, in fact. Country boy, city girl. A driver of a flash sports car versus a mud-splattered farm ute. Someone who much preferred having a fur child than the real thing.

But perhaps they had more in common than their chosen work.

Not that he wanted to compare memories of what it was like to lose a parent at an early age—any more than he'd want to talk about that failure of a marriage he'd had. He got the impression that Andi didn't want to talk about it, either, but he knew how interested his sometimes overly compassionate father could be in learning more.

'I'm so sorry,' Dave said. 'That's a terrible thing to have happened to you.' He shook his head. 'Those motorways around Auckland can be treacherous.'

'It was nowhere near Auckland,' Andi told him. 'I'd stopped at the place it happened on my way into Cutler's Creek. That's why I was on the road with Pingu when we met Jack and the sheep. There's still a cross there, down by the bridge.'

'Good heavens…' Dave sounded shocked. 'Were they on holiday here?'

'No. We lived not far from Queenstown. It was my grandmother who took me to live in Auckland. She was the only family I had left. I hadn't been back here since then.'

Jack was just as shocked as his father. No wonder she'd been distracted and hadn't been in total control of her dog on the road that day. And how hard had it been for her to come back to this part of the country in the first place? *Why* had she agreed to come?

He could sense that his father was wanting to ask the same questions.

Maybe he could do Andi a favour and stop her being forced to relive painful memories. Good grief, if anyone knew how that could reopen old wounds and make them bleed all over again, it should be him. Saving her from his father's well-meaning but possibly unwelcome questions might even go some way to making up for the way he'd treated her when they'd first met and she was probably trying to escape the ghosts of her own past.

'Talking about cute sheep,' he said. 'I was about to go and move my mob. Not along the road, just from one paddock to another. Why don't you come and help, Andi? There's enough daylight left to take the horses and a couple of dogs.' He dropped his gaze, hiding a smile. 'Not Pingu, though. Might be best if you leave him here with Dad.'

It was years since Andi had been riding. Not just riding but doing all the things that went with riding that she'd always enjoyed just as much.

Catching the pony and leading it to where it could be tied up. Brushing off any dried mud that caused discomfort under a saddle or girth. Picking hooves to get rid of stones. The tasks were all so familiar. The feel and smell of the huge, warm body. The friendly nudge from a nose trying to communicate the desire for that other piece of carrot still in her pocket.

Three farm dogs, including Bess, waited patiently while Jack took Andi into the barn to find a helmet that would fit her and collect the tack to put on the horses. He came to check her girth buckles were done up tightly enough when she'd put the saddle on Mary.

'Don't want any more accidents on my watch,' he murmured.

Then they were off, trotting down the side of the long driveway, clopping across the main road and then waiting for Jack to lean down from the back of Custard and open the wire gate to let them into the first, empty, paddock. It was dotted with tussock and flat enough near the road but became a slope further up that was going to turn into steeper, rockier ground which would be slower going. The dogs took off at a joyous run, Meg barking non-stop, heading for the next gate at the top of the hill, and Custard was bobbing his head, asking for a loose rein so he could also run.

Jack glanced back at Andi. 'You okay?'

'I'm good.' She knew how wide her smile was. She was loving this already.

Jack grinned back at her. 'Let's go, then…' He clicked his tongue, loosened his reins and Custard took off at a canter.

The little bay mare was not about to be left behind. She was smaller than Custard, so she ended up in a gallop as

Andi leaned forward to take her weight off the horse's back and let her really stretch her legs going up the hill. Jack looked over his shoulder. He was grinning again as it became a race.

'We'll call it a draw,' Jack said as they slowed down a short time later, but the look he gave Andi was impressed. 'You *can* ride, can't you?'

'A bit.'

Oh...he had that admiring look in his eyes again and that spear of sensation low down in her belly wasn't entirely because of any movement of the horse beneath her. They knew each other so much better now, too. They might have been successfully maintaining perfectly professional boundaries, but there were moments like this when Andi was reminded of what had been simmering between them from the moment they'd met.

She squeezed her legs against Mary and set off again. Another fast scramble uphill and a jump over a ditch was just the physical release she needed.

They were on the top of the hill within minutes and the view was spectacular. They could see the township of Cutler's Creek to one side, the patchwork of farmland and hills with the veins of a river and its tributaries running through it, and in the distance there was the glimpse of a mirror-still lake and the imposing peaks of the mountain ranges, including one that Andi never failed to recognise.

'Do you know why they were called the Remarkables?'

'Someone told me it was because the early settlers were sitting having a wine and admiring the sunset on the peaks and one of them said that they were remarkable.'

Andi laughed. 'I don't think the wine industry was up and running at that point. I heard it was because they're one of the only two mountain ranges on earth that run directly from north to south.'

'Where's the other one?'

'In the Rockies.' But Andi bit her lip. 'I might have to check that fact, though.'

'When you're not searching for cute sheep?'

Andi rolled her eyes. 'You're still offended, aren't you? Come on. Show me your sheep, then. I have to admit I didn't notice how cute they were when I first met them.'

Because she had been too busy noticing how cute the cowboy farmer was?

She'd put on a woollen jumper because it was cooler this evening, but Jack had his favourite black tee shirt on and bare arms. He hadn't gone for the kind of safety helmet she was wearing, either. He was wearing the cowboy hat that was so much a part of his look.

He wasn't just gorgeous looking, though, was he? He was…great company.

He was just like his dad. Two country men with big hearts and a range of skills that a city man could only dream of acquiring.

They were both vets as well, and Andi had seen and discussed enough of their work with them over the last week to know they were just as passionate about caring for animals as she was.

The difference between them was, while she really liked Dave Dunlop, it was his son, Jack, that she was fighting an attraction for.

And the more she learned about him, the harder it was becoming, because this was about so much more than looks or chemistry. He was a man who could be trusted. Admired, even. And that was blurring the well-defined boundaries of her comfort zone. Kind of like the way reconnecting with a place she'd never wanted to return to was also doing.

It was still possible to keep her emotions under control.

But it was disconcerting to feel them so much closer to the surface.

Jack was setting off to demonstrate all his admirable sheep-handling skills. How well he could ride, pivoting on the proverbial sixpence to change direction quickly, directing his dogs with whistles and calls, rounding the sheep into a tight, controlled mob and...

...and it was astonishingly sexy to watch him doing it.

Not that Andi had the time to simply watch. She was getting almost as many instructions as the dogs as they moved the sheep to another paddock where there was more feed. With Mary's help, Andi managed to keep up with the shifts of direction and speed changes that were required to keep the sheep moving steadily forward as a single unit.

She was quite out of breath by the time Jack latched the gate on the new paddock when all the sheep were safely contained. The dogs had jumped into a concrete trough full of water to cool down and Andi and Jack both dismounted to give the horses a bit of a rest.

They leaned on the gate to watch the sheep grabbing mouthfuls of the new grass.

'What's with the different coloured blobs of paint on their heads?' Andi asked.

'Blue blobs are the ones carrying twin lambs. I'll need to separate them out next week and give them some supplementary feed.'

'I can see a pink one, too. Over there...' Andi leaned a little closer to Jack as she pointed.

'Triplets. Sheep only have two teats so twins are easy,

but an extra one can be too much so we'll probably take one of them away to bottle raise.' He eyed Andi. 'I'll make sure it's a cute one and your wish will come true. It'll be all yours.'

Andi's eyes widened as she turned to catch his gaze and it was only then she realised quite how close they were standing.

'You said you wanted one.' Jack's voice was a sexy growl.

It felt like he was saying, *You said you wanted me*...

'Mmm...' The sound of agreement was slightly choked. Andi couldn't look away from him.

Something was changing, she could feel that, too. She knew she should try and stop it happening but...

...but she didn't want to.

This was...irresistible...

A silent conversation was happening between them. The flash of surprise in Jack's eyes morphed into something else.

Andi had no idea what messages she was sending because her brain was completely scrambled. She tried to shift her gaze but only succeeded in dropping it.

To Jack's lips. Just in time to see the one-sided curve of an appreciative smile fading as he bent his head.

To *kiss* her?

Andi's gaze flew up to see the question now in Jack's eyes.

Did she want this?

Andi couldn't summon any coherent words, but she was pretty sure that what she was thinking was written all over her face.

Hell, *yes*...

CHAPTER FIVE

'WHAT *IS* THAT?'

'Can't tell. It's been a bit chewed.' Jack shifted the tip of the endoscopy tube to get a better look at something that seemed partially embedded in the stomach of the young dog. 'Definitely plastic, which will be why it showed up better on ultrasound than X-ray. Oh...wait... are those *legs*?'

Andi leaned closer to peer at the screen as Jack paused to focus.

It was by far the closest she'd been to him since they'd been up on the hill an hour or so ago.

When he'd kissed her...

Oh, man...what *had* he been thinking?

He hadn't been thinking, that was the problem. He'd given in to an attraction that had been there from the get-go—despite him knowing perfectly well that it was a weakness he needed to keep well away from.

Not that it wasn't a great kiss. It had been an *astonishingly* good kiss, in fact. But he hadn't intended for it to happen, and while Andi had seemed perfectly happy to go along with the impulsive move, they'd both been a bit shocked afterwards, hadn't they?

One of the dogs—probably Bess—had given up her

soak in the trough and decided to stand right beside Jack as she shook herself vigorously and showered them both with a surprising volume of cold, dirty water. The kiss had been instantly broken, but something was still hanging in the air between them. He had no idea what, but they were both standing there staring at each other like stunned mullets.

Until his phone started ringing and he answered it to hear Dave telling him an emergency patient had turned up at the hospital.

It had been a relief to have that moment broken, though. To have something else that they could both focus on, along with the physical distraction of getting back on the horses and down the hill as quickly as it was safely possible.

'Sounds like an intestinal obstruction,' Jack told Andi as soon as they were on the way home. 'Adolescent dog, who's been off his food and vomiting for more than twenty-four hours now. Won't let anyone touch his abdomen and he's restless, so he's obviously in pain.'

'Do they have any idea what he might have eaten?'

'No. But Rufus has been a destructive pup. Staffy cross who gets bored when the kids are at school.'

They were silent as they cantered over the flat ground. Jack was slightly ahead of Andi and he was sure he could feel her gaze on his back. What was she thinking? Had *she* liked that kiss as much as he had?

Would she…maybe…want to do it again?

Not that he intended to find out. Even if he hadn't been grappling with unsettling ghosts from the past, having someone around who reminded him of his ex-wife, Jack could just imagine what his father would have to say if he found out that he was seducing their house guest. He needed to find something else to think about. Fast.

'What's the weirdest foreign object you've ever fished out of a dog?' he asked as he slowed to open the gate to cross the road.

'The end of a toilet brush. You?'

'Can't compete with that. I've had stones, a golf ball, hair ties and more than one case of a sock. Pair of undies, once.'

'I think that's up there with a toilet brush. I wonder what it'll be this time.'

'Let's just hope it doesn't need surgery. Don't know about you, but I'm starving…'

They'd delayed dinner to use the daylight still available to get the sheep moved, intending to eat as soon as they were done, but here they were and it was starting to look like it might be a while yet before they would get the chance to eat a meal.

'Yeah…' Andi sounded fascinated as she stared at the screen. 'Weird short legs. And that's an arm.'

'It'll be an action figure toy, I think. Looks vaguely familiar, in fact…'

'Do you think you can remove it endoscopically? Shall I find some rat tooth forceps or a net basket or a snare?'

'I'll try some grasping forceps, but I don't like the look of those sharp ends where it's been chewed. Causing a perforation will make things a whole lot worse.' And then he groaned. 'There's some bleeding here. I think there's a perforation already, so we might have to give up on a quick fix.'

'I'll let the family know. There's no point in them waiting here half the night.'

'Are you happy to do the anaesthetic? We can toss a coin if you'd rather do the surgery.'

'Your call,' Andi said. She was already moving towards the theatre door to get back to the anxious father and son who'd brought in their beloved family pet. 'I'm happy to do whatever you want me to.'

Oh...

No. No, no, no...

Jack wasn't even going to let himself think of anything unprofessional that he might be tempted to ask Andi to do.

He wasn't going to listen to that little voice in the back of his head that was suggesting that Andi was nothing at all like his ex-wife and anything that happened between them could only be the briefest of flings because she'd made no secret of how much she wanted to get back to the city.

His treacherous brain even came up with a new idea— that he might be able to get rid of those ghosts for good by having a good experience with someone like Andi. Maybe it would prove that the failure of his marriage hadn't been entirely his fault and he could finally let go and move on from the past.

No...

She was their locum.

They had to work together.

She was living in the same house as him. And his *father*...

It couldn't be allowed to happen.

No matter how much he might *want* to kiss her again.

On the way back to the clinic, Andi had convinced herself that kissing Jack had been a very bad idea and there was no way she wanted it to happen again.

Okay…maybe she'd had to argue with herself a little, when they'd been examining this unfortunate young dog—especially when his hands kept brushing hers when she was helping get the ultrasound and X-rays done—but the sensible side of her brain had won that argument.

Jack Dunlop was so far out of her comfort zone when it came to men that he hadn't been a contender to *kiss*, let alone to allow it to happen again or, heaven help her, go any further.

Because he was dangerous.

He made her feel things that she didn't want to feel. That perhaps the physical attraction was too strong. That, even if you had no intention of letting it happen, you could fall in love with a man like Jack Dunlop. Emotions—especially intense ones like love—were dangerous because they had the power to destroy your world. She needed to stay in control.

Because that was the only way to stay safe.

Andi wasn't quite sure how it had happened, but she managed to put it out of her mind completely as they began the more serious task of operating on this patient. She induced the anaesthetic in the already well-sedated dog, ensuring the drugs were mixed according to predetermined concentrations and the parameters on the anaesthetic equipment would be delivering adequate oxygen, ventilation and breathing rates, and then she shaved the belly, disinfected it and positioned Rufus on his back while Jack was getting scrubbed in. It would have been useful to have another assistant, but the retractor Jack employed to keep the surgical field open and visible was almost as good.

It was only a very short time ago that Andi had seen his hands engaged in farmer-type activities, like throwing a saddle onto a horse or tightening girth buckles, opening gate latches or chopping dog roll to feed his pack in a hurry. They looked like someone else's hands now, towards the opposite end of a spectrum that measured precision, encased in sterile gloves and handling surgical instruments, like scalpels and forceps, with a skill that let Andi relax and simply watch.

Bad move, she decided, only moments later. Because her gaze was still on his hands and she was thinking of something else she'd seen him doing with them earlier this evening. Or, rather, she'd felt them.

She could *still* feel the way he'd cupped her chin between his finger and thumb—a relaxed version of how he held them in his mouth when whistling at his dogs—as he'd lowered his mouth to touch hers. She'd been just as aware of the touch of his fingers as the way his lips were moving over hers. She had wanted those fingers to move towards other parts of her body, hadn't she? And then she'd felt the touch of his tongue against hers and lost the ability to think coherently at all, until they'd been showered with that icy water from the trough, thanks to Bess. The shock had sent them jerking apart, but there had been a moment then, when they'd simply stared at each other and there was an intensity in that eye contact that was…

…something that Andi had never felt before in her life.

She was still watching his hands as he located the foreign object this dog had swallowed. She picked up a kidney dish to receive whatever it was, but there was nothing more she needed to do until she could assist Jack in what needed to be done in the way of repairs and closing the wound. She could hear the steady tick of the heart monitor and see that all the dog's vital signs were reassuringly normal, so it wasn't a problem that her brain was taking advantage of a momentary lull in the need to focus to the total exclusion of anything else.

Was it trying to revive the argument that had already been dealt with? Offering that curiosity about how she'd felt in the wake of that kiss as a reason she might want to let it happen again?

What if that totally new feeling wasn't something to run away from?

What if it was something important that she hadn't known was missing from her life?

Would it, perhaps, be a good idea to spend some more time alone with Jack?

'Ah *ha*…' Jack's tone suggested a lightbulb moment— as if he knew the answer to the questions flitting through Andi's head. He was even nodding his agreement, which gave Andi a frisson of something that felt almost like excitement.

But, no…he was far more professionally focused than she was right now. 'I know what this is,' he told Andi.

'Oh…?'

'I had one of these when I was a kid—back in the nineties. It was a promotion at petrol stations. Not toys as much as collectors' items to celebrate famous All Blacks.' The plastic blob dropped into the kidney dish Andi was holding with a solid thud. 'I seem to remember that this one was the most sought after.'

Andi peered at the object. A figurine with an oversized head, wearing a black shirt and shorts.

'It's Jonah Lomu,' Jack prompted. He shook his head. 'You're not into rugby?'

'Not really, no…'

'Someone will want that back. They might be a bit upset that his legs have been amputated below the knees, but that doesn't necessarily mean it can't trump your toilet brush, does it?'

'Not at all. You totally deserve first prize.'

Andi could hear the smile in Jack's voice. She could see the crinkles at the corners of his eyes. She could feel it again, too. That odd feeling, whatever it was, in the way his gaze was holding hers—as if he could see right into her soul.

She didn't like that.

What if he saw what her grandmother had seen?

That she wasn't worth admiring, let alone loving?

That he'd been right in not wanting her to be here in the first place?

The thought was disturbing enough to make it easy to break the eye contact. Besides, it was time to check their patient's vital signs again.

'Okay…' Jack cleared his throat. 'Let's get this perforation repaired and then we'll give the whole field a thorough flush to get it as clean as possible and we can close up.'

But he looked up again a moment later. 'Speaking of first prizes…do you want to come to the dog trials this weekend? They need a vet there, but I'll be able to concentrate a lot better when I'm competing if I know someone's keeping an eye on Dad and making sure he's not overdoing things on his first outing since the accident.'

This invitation wasn't an opportunity to be alone with Jack. She'd be in a crowd of people, with his dad as a chaperone, so she was perfectly safe—from any intentions that either of them might have to repeat that kiss.

Andi had never been to a dog trial before. It was always worth trying something different, wasn't it? You might just discover a passion you didn't know you had. Or you could cross it off the list of things that you wanted in your life and try something else instead.

'Sure,' she found herself saying. 'Can Pingu come?'

Pingu was absolutely fascinated by the dog trials.

He sat by Andi's feet, bolt upright, quivering with the excitement of the crowd of spectators, the constant barking of the huntaways and watching the dogs working with the sheep.

Andi, who was keeping a very tight hold on Pingu's leash, was just as fascinated and was grateful to have Dave standing beside her and explaining what was going on while the competitors and their dogs were on the course.

'So this is the zigzag hunt for huntaways. You need a nice, steep hill like this and the three sheep get released at the bottom and the dog has to get them up the zigzag course between those markers and through the gap between those two gates at the top of the hill. The dog has to always face the sheep and not the handler. That's why they're called huntaways—they're sending the sheep away from the handler. Heading dogs bring the sheep towards the handler.'

'Oh…it's Jack's turn. Look…'

'Wouldn't be surprised if Meg wins this with Jed out of the picture. All depends on how cooperative the sheep feel like being, mind you. The bolshy ones can be impossible. One of them will make a run for it and the others just follow.'

Andi might not be quivering, but she was watching

Jack as intently as Pingu was, listening to his whistles and calls, holding her breath as Meg drove the sheep through the first set of markers and then made them change direction. He looked absolutely at home, standing tall and confident in his jeans and gumboots and the signature red-and-black-checked bush shirt of a man who loved to be outdoors. He even held a shepherd's crook and Andi found herself watching him rather than the progress of the sheep up the hill.

Thinking about that kiss…

When the run ended and the clapping and whistles from spectators suggested that Jack and Meg had done very well, Andi watched Meg, clearly not slowed down by her pregnancy, flying back down the hill in response to Jack's whistle. She coiled her body around Jack's legs, waving her tail and looking up at him adoringly, and Andi found herself smiling as Jack leaned down and gave her some love, ruffling the hair on her head and patting her back. She could feel the bond between man and dog even from this distance. Being kind to dogs was…

…well, it was pretty damned sexy, that's what it was.

Everybody knew everybody here and it seemed that the whole community wanted to talk to Dave and Jack. Maureen arrived and insisted that Dave rested for a while. She took him away to sit in the ute and eat sausages wrapped in bread from the sausage sizzle being provided as a fundraiser for a local charity. Andi wasn't left alone, though. She'd only been in the district for a short time, but she didn't feel like a stranger. She recognised some people who'd come through the vet clinic and Terry was here with Jed, who was wearing his knee support.

'I'll put him back in the truck in a minute,' Terry said.

'Thought I'd come and watch Jack and Bess in the short head and yard.'

'The what?'

'It's a heading dog class—dog has to drive the sheep along a marked track, through hurdles and then get them into the pen. The only thing the handler's allowed to do to help is to hold the gate of the pen open. They get up to fourteen minutes, but I've seen Jack and Bess do it in less than seven.'

Seven minutes.

It wasn't a long time, but it would be long enough.

Too long, really, if she was going to be staring at Jack Dunlop and thinking about that kiss. Feeling those delicious spears of sensation that started deep in her belly and spread like liquid fire through her body every time she remembered what it was like when his lips had touched hers.

The more she thought about it, the more Andi was convincing herself that she wanted it to happen again. To find out if it was as good as the first time. To see if it would go any further. To find out what she might have been missing in avoiding the kind of man she had always assumed would be totally unsuitable?

She'd said it herself, after all.

Whatever the outcome, the learning experience you got almost always made it worth trying something different.

Jack dipped the gauze into the antiseptic solution and gently cleaned around one of the pins attaching the halo brace to his father's skull. Then he used another piece to dry the skin.

'Looking good, Dad. The skin's not red or oozy. Have you got any pain?'

'Bit of a headache, but I've been on my feet for a lot longer today.'

'I should have got Maureen to take you home early.'

'And miss out on seeing you getting all those ribbons?' Dave's smile was weary but happy. 'It's been a great day. I think Andi enjoyed it as much as we did. Pingu certainly did. I think he got more attention than any of the working dogs. Every kid there had to come and pat him.'

Jack grunted. They might have been enjoying themselves, but the fact that people had noticed them so much was because it was obvious they were out of place on a high country farm. They wouldn't get a second glance if they were sitting in a trendy café in a big city.

No…that wasn't true. Andi would get a second glance anywhere, especially from men. He'd noticed a few going in her direction at the trials today. Someone needed to warn those young farmers not to even think about it. Those city girls might fall in love with a country boy and be quite prepared to embrace the challenge of living in the middle of nowhere, but they'd get bored soon enough and fall out of love with everything, including them, and life would get miserable for everybody.

Like his life had been.

It had felt like it was his fault. He couldn't live in a city. He couldn't make his wife happy in the country. Being with him was never going to be enough.

He was never going to be enough.

It was no wonder he'd avoided getting too involved with anyone again for a long, long time. If he didn't stay with anyone too long, they couldn't find out that he was a failure when it came to something long term.

'Are you done?' Dave's voice broke into his thoughts.

'Yep.'

'Good. I still need to clean my teeth and Andi's probably back from her walk now. She'll be wanting to have a shower, I expect, after being out on the farm all day.'

Jack didn't want to think about Andi having a shower.

Standing naked under a rain of hot water. With maybe a cascade of shampoo bubbles streaming down her bare back…

Oh, *man*…was he ever going to get that kiss out of his head?

He had to make an effort to tune back into what his father was saying.

'The cottage?'

'That's what I said. Andi's not about to rush back to Auckland, but I reckon she'd appreciate a bit more of her own space.'

Her own space?

Away from the house? And his father?

A…private space?

Dave's voice was just a background to his thoughts. 'I might wander down tomorrow and see if anything needs doing to make it habitable after those shearers used it last.'

'I can do that.' Jack actually needed to shake his head to clear it. 'I'll go down when you're in bed. I want to make sure Meg didn't overdo it today. That litter of pups isn't too far away.'

He took some of the roast chicken left over from dinner to Meg as a treat and made sure she had a comfortable nest of blankets in her kennel. He'd move her up to the house soon and she could live in the laundry room while she raised her babies. It might put Bess's nose out of joint because she was the only farm dog who got to live up at the house, but she'd stopped growling at Pingu a while back now. She'd even let the little dog sit beside her when they were watching others compete today.

Had Pingu seen that as a thawing in their relationship? Was that why he bounced out of the shadows of the barn as Jack and Bess headed away from the kennels?

Bess froze, her head lowering as if she was on the case of a disobedient sheep.

'Easy, girl,' Jack murmured.

Andi appeared from around the corner of the barn as well. The moonlight was doing something interesting to her blonde hair, making it silver rather than gold. Jack had to squash another image of it being full of soap suds.

He cleared his throat. 'You two are having a long walk tonight.'

'We've been working,' Andi told him. 'I think Pingu wants to learn to be a sheepdog. We've been practising going right and left.'

'You might want to make that "over" for left and "away" for right,' Jack suggested. 'Then you'll sound more like you know what you're talking about.'

'I'll need to learn to whistle, too.' Andi put her fingers to her lips and blew on them but made no sound.

Jack laughed. 'You're such a girl.'

Andi's jaw dropped. 'You can't say things like that.'

Jack was still grinning. 'I used to get away with it in primary school.'

It looked as if Andi was having difficulty stifling a smile. 'I'll bet you did…'

Jack held her gaze. 'But we're grown-ups now, so I suppose I should apologise for saying that.'

She wasn't looking away. And something was changing. There was an undercurrent to the banter that was making Jack wonder if she was thinking about that kiss.

Because he sure as hell was…

It was going to happen again.

Jack was about to kiss her and that melty thing was out of control. It was even affecting important structures— like her knee joints? Good grief…was she actually going weak at the knees?

Something was certainly becoming weak and it wasn't just the muscles she needed to use to break that eye contact. Andi had the horrible suspicion that it was any will-power she might need to summon in order to stop this kiss happening. Neither could she stop the flash coming from the part of her brain that was most definitely not the sensible side.

Jack's right, it was telling her. You're both grown up. *You're allowed to kiss him…* And then, even worse—*You know you want to…*

It would be the heart ruling the head. Not going to happen.

Why not? You're not going to marry the guy. Or even fall in love with him. This is just like a holiday.

It would be totally unprofessional.

Not working hours now, is it?

The voice faded as Jack's face came closer. This was a *déjà vu* moment now. Except she wasn't leaning on a farm gate while it was still daylight. The darkness and privacy of the night was surrounding them and it was cold enough to make that first touch of Jack's lips as hot as flames.

Andi had the answer to her question instantly. This

kiss was just as good as the first one. But then it deepened to another level as the loose grip of Jack's hands on
her shoulders tightened and he pulled her close enough
for her whole body to be touching his.

Dear *Lord*...

Andi did make an attempt to regain control—as soon
as she could take a breath—but it was undermined by
how indecisive her voice sounded.

'We shouldn't be doing this.'

Was Jack *smiling* at her?

'Don't you want to?'

Andi tried to say 'no' but the word wouldn't come out.

'Who's going to know?' he murmured.

'Your father, for one.' Andi pulled in a breath. This
might work. 'And he might tell his mate Warren, who
might change his mind about offering me a partnership
due to my unprofessional conduct, and...and that partnership is something I really, really want. It's the only reason
I agreed to come here.'

Jack shrugged. 'There's no reason for anyone to know.
Including Dad.'

'We're living in the same house.'

'Ah...' One of Jack's eyebrows rose. 'That's why I'm
out here. Dad thought you might like to have your own
space, so I'm going to check the shearer's cottage to see
if it's up to scratch.'

He wasn't smiling at her now. He was, however, holding her gaze with an intensity that sent a shiver down
Andi's spine.

'Come with me,' he said softly. 'We'll check it out together and see how good it might be. Not that it has to be
perfect. I mean...it's not forever, is it? You could try it just

for a night or two, and if it doesn't suit, we'll never need to mention it again. Or you could enjoy it for the rest of your time here. Entirely your choice. No pressure.'

Andi's breath had caught somewhere in her chest and wasn't going anywhere. Jack wasn't talking about her using the cottage, was he? He was talking about exactly what she'd been thinking about far too much.

Finding out what it would be like to be with someone she would never remotely consider being with in her normal life.

Part of Andi's brain was registering that this was a once-in-a-lifetime opportunity. How many cowboys was she likely to meet in her future in Auckland? The question was, how much could she really trust Jack Dunlop?

Then she remembered the bond she had sensed between Jack and his father. She thought of the way his dogs looked up at him and the way he'd ruffled Bess's hair when she'd done a good job today.

And there was the answer to that question.

She could absolutely trust Jack.

Andi could breathe again. And speak.

'Yes, please...' she whispered. 'I *would* like to see the cottage.'

CHAPTER SIX

JACK HAD ALMOST forgotten that Andi owned a pair of white jeans.

She'd even taken his advice and purchased a pair of bright blue, long-sleeved overalls a few days ago—at the farm and rural supplies store in Cutler's Creek. She had them on for the first time today and Jack had to wonder how she managed to make such a shapeless item of clothing look sexy. He watched her tucking the legs of the overalls into her black gumboots with the red band on the top.

Jack grinned at her over the open door of his ute that he was leaning on. Not that he could tell her how sexy she looked. Not during working hours, anyway.

'You almost look like a country vet,' he said.

'I feel like one,' Andi said. 'Now that you're finally letting me go on a farm job.' She looked into the back seat of the double cab. 'Bess is coming?'

'Yep. Always comes with me.'

Andi gave him a look.

Jack lifted his eyebrows. 'You want the penguin dog to come?'

She lifted her eyebrows right back at him. 'Why not?'

'Because he might cause havoc.'

'Not if he's anywhere near Bess. You know he just sits

there and stares at her. He's started copying everything she does. I think he's totally smitten...'

Jack sighed. 'Go and get him, then. But be quick. Marigold is not feeling very well.'

Her awkward running in her gumboots made him smile. She looked like a kid playing dress-ups. But Jack knew just how unchildlike Andrea Chamberlain could be. He had, in fact, discovered a whole new level of adult fun in the old shearer's cottage the other night in a sexual encounter that had left him...

...blindsided, to be honest.

The sheer *heat* of the woman. And that captivating mix that was somehow vulnerable but brave and adventurous at the same time had left him wishing he'd slowed things down a whole heap more and made it last as long as possible.

They'd crept back into the house quietly and Dave didn't show any signs of suspecting anything untoward had been going on at breakfast time the next morning.

'Jack tells me he showed you the cottage.'

Andi looked as if she was swallowing her bite of toast rather hurriedly.

'What did you think of it?'

'I liked it.' Andi's smile had been the picture of innocence, but Jack knew she'd been avoiding catching his gaze. 'It's a bit of Central Otago history with that stonework and the old fireplace, isn't it?'

'You make it yours, then.' Dave nodded. 'And enjoy it while you're here.'

Jack had enjoyed it again himself, a day or two later, when the cottage had had a spring clean, thanks to Maureen, and there was fresh linen on the bed, but if he was really honest, nothing was going to beat that first time—when everything had been a bit dusty and deserted and they'd made love on a bare mattress with the moonlight sneaking in through a grimy window.

He'd been completely wrong about Andi being a princess, hadn't he?

She didn't seem to have been at all put off by that dusty room and bare mattress.

'You'd better behave,' Andi whispered to Pingu when she released him from his working hours' crate in the back of the animal hospital and clipped on his harness. 'This is the first farm callout I've been allowed to go on and I want...'

Her voice trailed into silence as they got outside and hurried back to the ute. She couldn't say it out loud. Imagine if Jack knew that what she really wanted to happen today was that he would be impressed at how she could cope with being out of her comfort zone.

Not just with potentially doing surgery away from a well-equipped and hygienic operating theatre in a veterinary hospital. She wanted him to be as impressed with her as she was with him.

Who knew that such a confident, masculine guy who was perfectly at ease wrangling horses and dogs and sheep and could whistle like a pro even without using a shepherd's whistle or his fingers could be so...*gentle* in bed? Considerate. Exciting. Sheer, irrepressible *fun*?

Andi had had no idea what she'd been missing out on.

That the feeling of being wanted, even if it was purely in a physical sense, was a very powerful thing.

Wanted. Appreciated. *Loved*, even, for those magic minutes together when nothing and nobody else existed.

She did know how unlikely it was she was going to find anybody like Jack back in Auckland, mind you.

And that was her excuse for behaving so out of character while she was here. She was going to jolly well make the most of her time with Jack Dunlop. She wanted him to remember her for more than their personal connection out of work hours, however. She wanted him to send back a glowing reference to Warren to make sure he didn't forget about that partnership offer.

So, here she was, on a visit out to a farm to see a house cow by the name of Marigold and she was trying hard to retrieve everything she'd learned at vet school about treating health issues with ruminants. She suspected that Jack might find it amusing to throw her in at the deep end.

She wasn't wrong. He parked the ute with all their gear in the back beside the pen where the farmer, Glenys, was waiting for them.

'This is Andi,' he told Glenys. 'She's going to take a look at Marigold for you.'

Andi was already looking at Marigold, who was a beautiful example of a Jersey cow, with huge brown eyes and a face that advertised how gentle she was likely to be.

'We hand milk her,' Glenys told Andi. 'She's off her food and her milk production has dropped right off.'

Andi rubbed Marigold's nose. 'Has anything else changed for her? Has she had a calf recently?'

'Yes. We've got the baby shut in the barn so it didn't get in the way. I think Marigold's relieved to have a break from it trying to feed. I'm thinking we might need to start bottle-feeding the baby.'

Andi could feel Jack watching her as she made a visual assessment of their patient, although he was trying to look like a casual observer as he stooped and picked a long stalk of grass. From the corner of her eye, Andi could see Bess watching from the back window of the ute. And yeah… Pingu had to be standing on his back legs for his head to get into the frame of the window. Glenys was holding Marigold's halter and she was watching intently.

'We all love Marigold,' she said, with a catch in her voice. 'We've had her since she was a calf and she's a part of the family. The kids would be absolutely devastated if anything happened to her.'

No pressure, then, Andi thought. Not that she really felt on her own here. Jack might be giving her the space to show what she could do, but she knew she could trust him to jump in if she asked for assistance.

It was obvious that Marigold wasn't distressed by being separated from her calf, which suggested her behaviour wasn't normal. Andi also noted the asymmetry in the cow's abdomen when she looked at her from the back. She ran her hands over Marigold's belly and then put her stethoscope against the skin and began to percuss the abdomen by flicking her fingers against it firmly. She could hear the distinct pinging sound like hitting a metal drum on the left side.

'I think she's got an LDA,' she told Glenys.

'A what?'

'A left displaced abomasum. It's the cow's fourth stomach. It gets filled with gas, floats up like a balloon and moves to the left side.'

Jack was chewing on the end of the stalk of grass. He was also nodding. 'I could hear the ping from here,' he said.

'Can it be treated?' Glenys asked. 'Is it dangerous?'

'It can be dangerous,' Andi said. 'But it's treatable.'

'With surgery,' Jack confirmed. 'We make an incision in the right flank, find what feels like a basketball on the left side, let the air out and pull the stomach back into its correct position. We can stitch it into place and make sure it doesn't happen again.'

'Goodness me…' Glenys put her forehead against Marigold's neck. 'That sounds major.'

'You might be surprised,' Jack said reassuringly. 'I've seen cows walk off and start grazing as soon as they're stitched up. She's going to feel so much better when this is sorted.' He dropped the stalk of grass and caught Andi's gaze. 'I'll get us set up for surgery, shall I?'

Marigold wasn't the only one who felt a lot better when the surgery was over. Andi was breathing a huge sigh of relief that it had all gone without a hitch.

So was Glenys. She watched Andi putting in the final stitches to close the incision.

'That's so neat,' she said. 'And it's not bothering Marigold at all.'

'The local hasn't worn off yet, but she'll be fine. Keep an eye on it and let us know if you notice any discharge or swelling.'

'Thank you so much, Andi. I'd heard you were good. Terry's been singing your praises after you operated on Jed.' She glanced at Jack. 'How's Dave doing?'

'Getting there. He'll have to keep the brace on for a few weeks longer and will still need to be careful when it comes off, but his medical team is happy with the way he's healing.'

'So you might need Andi to hang around for a while

yet, then?' Glenys smiled at Andi as she snipped off the last stitch. 'Dave might want to slow down enough to retire one of these days.'

Jack shook his head. 'You're barking up the wrong tree there, Glenys. Andi here's a city girl through and through. She had to have her arm twisted to come here in the first place and I'm quite sure she's hanging out to get back to Auckland.'

Andi had done a neat job, but she found herself frowning as she gave the wound a final check and then sprayed it with a liquid bandage to help keep it clean. Jack was right, of course. She *was* hanging out to get back to Auckland. To her chic apartment close to the waterfront that afforded a spectacular view of the harbour. It was right in the heart of New Zealand's most vibrant city with limitless choice of amazing restaurants and bars and venues for sought-after internationally acclaimed concerts and shows. She had beautiful parks to go walking in with Pingu and countless beaches within easy reach. And she *was* missing her yoga classes and her personal trainer and taking Pingu for a puppaccino at her favourite café.

So why did it feel vaguely hurtful that Jack sounded so cheerful about her wanting to get away from Cutler's Creek?

He hadn't given the impression that he was hanging out for her to disappear back to the big smoke the last time he'd come to visit her in the cottage, that was for sure. She'd been left feeling as if he would be happy to be sharing her bed for quite some time to come.

As happy as she was to have him there?

It wasn't that she was really hurt, of course. They both knew this was just a bit of a fling. Something to help pass the time before she went back where she belonged. An interlude before Jack got down to the serious business of finding the nice country girl who would be happy to give him that large tribe of children he wanted in his future. They were such complete opposites, it could only ever be a fling.

A sexual thing.

The old friendship with benefits kind of thing.

So why did it feel as if there was something lurking beneath the surface that shouldn't be there?

Why did it make Andi feel as if they shouldn't be doing it at all, even though she didn't want to be the one to pull the plug?

It was going to end anyway, wasn't it?

'There…' Andi put the spray can of liquid bandage back into the box of gear. 'I think we're all done here.' She went to pick up the box, but Jack beat her to it.

'I've got it. You can't do all the work.' His smile was lazy. 'Word might get around the district and someone will start a petition to persuade you to stay in Cutler's Creek.'

He walked away towards the ute and, for some reason, it was an effort not to watch him. She bent to pick up a crumpled glove and some discarded packaging instead.

Glenys was untying Marigold, but she was also watching Jack. 'Shame you're not going to be staying that much longer,' she said. She seemed to be giving Andi the ghost of a wink as she looked up. 'Must be a breath of fresh air for those Dunlop men to have a woman around for a while. Might have even been enough to persuade one of them to move on.'

'Move on?'

'Dave's never got over losing Jack's mum, but everyone

can see that he and Maureen would be great together. And as for Jack…' Glenys shook her head. 'It's been nearly ten years. More than enough time to get over it.'

Andi raised her eyebrows, but Marigold was pulling Glenys towards a patch of long, green grass. She was obviously feeling better enough to realise she was hungry, which was a good sign. Glenys looked back over her shoulder.

'Yeah…' she said quietly. 'Just because his marriage didn't work out doesn't mean he has to stay single for the rest of his life, does it?'

It was very quiet.

Jack could only hear the engine noise of the ute and the sound of the thick tread of his all-terrain tyres on the unsealed farm road.

If he glanced over his shoulder, he could see two happy dogs sitting on the back seat, the windows cracked enough to give them some fresh air, but only Bess was tall enough to reach the gap with her nose. If he looked sideways, he could see Andi's profile. That cute snubbed nose and a shorter wisp of hair that had escaped from her ponytail to curl in front of her ear.

She was looking straight ahead through the windscreen and there was something about her body language that suggested she was deep in thought.

'Penny for them?'

She flicked him a glance but didn't say anything.

'You've never done that particular surgery before, have you?'

Andi shook her head.

'You did a good job.'

'Only because you talked me through it. I probably wouldn't have remembered to make the incision on the opposite side and then reach in like that to find the stomach. Or where the best spot to attach it was.'

She'd done it, though. The expression on her face when she had her arm, in a full-length surgical sleeve, right inside Marigold as she concentrated on piercing the distended organ to release the pressure of air had been worth seeing. That sheer determination to do the best job she possibly could was pretty impressive.

'You did a good job,' Jack repeated. 'What does it matter if I was talking you through it? You won't need me next time.'

They both fell silent for a beat.

They both knew how unlikely it was that there would be a next time.

Andi got out to open the farm gate to the main road but avoided looking at Jack as she got back into the vehicle.

Okay…something was off. Ever since that first time in the cottage—no, ever since that first kiss—there'd been something hanging in the air between them. He'd really thought that nothing could beat that first time they'd made love on that bare mattress in the dusty cottage but, unbelievably, each time was better than the one before. They were getting familiar with each other's bodies. Physically comfortable enough with each other that the sex was… well, it was off-the-charts good, that's what it was.

And whatever it was in the air was thick enough to almost be something he could touch. Some kind of electricity? It certainly felt like sparks, that's for sure. Even a heartbeat of eye contact was enough to be able to feel them and… Jack liked it. A lot. They made him feel increasingly more alive as they built up the anticipation to when he and Andi could be alone together again.

But they were alone right now and…he couldn't feel the sparks.

Had Andi flicked a switch and turned them off for some reason?

Had she been offended that he'd talked her through that surgery?

Or…wait…

'I didn't offend you, did I?' he asked. 'By telling Glenys that you were hanging out to get back to the big smoke?'

'Why would I be?' Andi was looking out of her side window now. 'It's true.'

The road was empty both in front and behind them. They were a fair distance out of Cutler's Creek, with acres of sheep-dotted farmland around them and a wall of mountains ahead. There was a wide enough shoulder on the road to pull off and that's what Jack did, without even thinking about it.

'Why are we stopping?' Andi asked. 'Is something wrong?'

'You tell me.'

Andi met the steady look he was giving her. For a moment, he thought she was going to do that thing that women are so good at doing and claim there was nothing wrong when it was clear there was, but she didn't.

'You never told me you were married,' she said.

Jack's jaw dropped. 'I'm not.'

'But you *were.*'

'Ancient history. What the hell has that got to do with anything?'

Andi looked disconcerted now. 'I don't know... I guess... I thought we were friends, Jack.'

'We are.' He tried a smile. 'I never go to bed with someone I don't like.'

His humour fell like a lead balloon.

'Did Glenys say something?'

'Yes. She said it was time you moved on.' Andi tucked that stray curl behind her ear. 'She's got a point, you know. You need to be getting on with it, if you want that tribe of kids you said you wanted. Unless you think you're going to get lucky and have triplets, like that sheep of yours.'

Her attempt at humour was even worse than his, so Jack ignored it, but she did have a point.

'Maybe I'll adopt some,' he said. 'And bump the numbers up that way.'

Andi was silent and Jack mentally kicked himself. She'd been orphaned at a young age. Could the idea of adoption have touched a nerve that might still be raw even after so many years? No...she'd been miffed well before his ill-considered comment.

'I don't get why you're upset,' he said. 'Why does it even matter that I've had a marriage that didn't work out?'

'I'm not upset. I'm just...surprised, I guess.'

'That anyone would have wanted to marry me?'

'No...' At least that made her smile. And then she looked serious again. 'Maybe I'm surprised that it didn't work out. You're a nice guy, Jack.' She lifted an eyebrow. 'I'd give you a good reference.'

Jack gave a huff of laughter. 'I'll keep that in mind.' Then he let his breath out in a sigh. 'I didn't tell you I'd been married because it's something I prefer not to think about. I met Roz in Queenstown when I was fresh out of vet school. She was an event planner and she was good at it. The bigger the better, but she said she was happy to give it all up for love and become a rural vet's wife. Until she wasn't happy, which was pretty much after the honeymoon was over and she found out what living in a small, country town was like. We stuck it out for a year—even tried living in the city for a while—but it was unbearable for both of us and the only way out was to go our separate ways. Hers was off to New York to get back together with the man she'd broken up with to be with me.'

'*Ouch…*' Andi visibly winced. 'Sorry…'

'Wasn't your fault.'

'I'm sorry I made you talk about it.'

Jack shrugged. 'It was bound to come up. Everybody knows too much about you in a place like Cutler's Creek. They've been watching me for years, waiting for me to move on, but…it just makes it less likely when I know I'm being watched.'

'I'm not watching.'

Jack laughed. 'No…you're *being* watched. That's why I told Glenys that you're only around for a short time before you escape back to the city.' He caught her gaze. 'I like what we have,' he added quietly. 'And it's not going to be for much longer, so I'd prefer to keep it private.'

Andi was holding his gaze. 'I like it, too,' she said.

Jack was smiling again.

They were back. Those sparks. So thick in the confines of this vehicle cab that he could almost taste them.

He could even see them dancing in Andi's eyes. All was right in the world again. He loosened his seat belt and leaned towards her. A kiss was definitely called for here, wasn't it?

Just to seal the deal and make sure things were back to normal.

CHAPTER SEVEN

THE DAYS WERE flying past as the spring workload ramped up.

On top of routine farm and clinic work and dealing with emergencies, there were baby animals everywhere. Calves had been arriving since the end of winter, there were foals and baby goats and kittens being born and lambing season was well underway.

The days were long and the weather changeable—warm one day, pouring with rain the next, windy enough to be blowing the blossom off fruit trees and there was even the threat of a late snowfall to worry about.

Andi was wearing an oilskin raincoat and her gumboots as she helped Jack move his sheep into a paddock behind the woolshed as daylight was fading. They hadn't taken the horses this time because it was the end of a long day and it was starting to rain, so the sooner they got the job done, the better.

Jack was driving his all-terrain vehicle, which was like a four-wheeled motorbike with a wide enough seat for two people and it had a tray at the back that the dogs could sit on. They had Bess and Jazz with them. Meg was due to produce her own babies soon and was back at the house with Pingu and Dave, who was mobile enough now to be preparing dinner.

The bench seat of the quad bike was quite a snug fit for two people, but Andi didn't mind at all being close enough for her leg to be pressed against Jack's. It was her job to jump out and open and close the gates and she was getting cold enough to be increasingly grateful for the warmth of his body.

Okay…it wasn't just because it was cold.

She loved being this close to Jack.

Who would have thought—when she was so horrified at Warren's decree that she should go and work in his mate's rural vet practice and live on a farm for *months*— that she could be out in all weathers like this and doing the kind of veterinary or farm work she had never been attracted to and…that she would end up enjoying it?

Not that Andi wasn't looking forward to getting back to her predictable, safe routine in the city and her clean, dry working conditions. If anything, she was going to appreciate them more for having experienced such a contrast.

Would she appreciate being amongst the kind of men she'd always considered predictable and safe as well? Men who didn't give or demand a level of emotional involvement that could threaten the safe boundaries of a life she had painstakingly built for herself. Men who were nothing at all like Jack Dunlop. But that was what made them safe, wasn't it?

Andi wasn't so sure about that part of her return to her old life. She was trying not to think about it, in fact, other than that it was the perfect excuse to make the most of this never-to-be-repeated blip in her career trajectory.

The stolen times with Jack, that only they knew about,

were setting a bar in her sex life that was very unlikely to ever be available again. To be honest, Andi had believed that physical chemistry like this only happened between the pages of a book or in a movie, not in real life.

Was it all that practice Jack had had as a bad boy that made him so attuned to discovering anything and everything that could make a woman whimper in pleasure?

Or was it because it was almost illicit, given that she was here in a purely professional capacity as a favour to the man who had the power to give her the career she'd always dreamed of?

Or that she would never have considered getting in this deep when it would have been an instant deal-breaker to discover that a man she was dating wanted to have a big family?

No…she knew that there was some strange alchemy that was making this…*friendship*…with Jack Dunlop so extraordinary. She had stepped out of her real life, which meant that she could pretend to be someone different. Someone who didn't have the shackles of having to make sure she didn't do anything that could undermine the security of the future she was building for herself?

Yes…this was the opportunity to try anything and everything she'd never dared to try before and she only had to remind herself that the window of time was closing fast to find the courage to do exactly that.

She blinked raindrops off her eyelashes and tried to focus on the task at hand.

'Are we going down the driveway or through the horse paddock on the way back?'

'Down the driveway. There's a gate between your cottage and the woolshed. That's the paddock with the best macrocarpa shelter belt.' He threw her a grin. 'I'll leave a supply of lamb coats with you. You'll be able to see any new arrivals out your window and you can get their coats on as soon as they're born.'

'Coats? *Really*?'

'Really. I've got commercial plastic or felt models, but the best are the ones that Maureen and her "knit and natter" club make.'

Andi laughed at the thought of a group of women knitting coats for lambs, but Jack gave her a stern look.

'Low temperatures, freezing rain and wind chill are dangerous. Hypothermia's the biggest killer for newborn lambs. I know they've got their mums and that good, thick hedge there, but Maureen's coats are very cute and...' His voice was as warm as his smile. 'I like to look after my babies.'

Andi climbed off the seat to open the gate. There was a brave bunch of daffodils blooming beside the gate post, which gave her enough pleasure to make up for how hard it was to get the hook through the ring and release the gate when her fingers were half frozen. The dogs jumped off the quad bike, ready to streak ahead once they got into the paddock where the sheep were huddled, their backs to the wind.

She watched Jack, standing up behind the wheel as he drove the bike through the gate.

He would look after his own babies with even more devotion than any newborn lambs, wouldn't he? She could imagine him in ten years' time with a few of his kids—adopted or biological—squashed onto the bike's seat beside him, eager to be out on the farm helping their dad with another lambing season.

The mother of those children was out there some-where. Probably not that far away given Jack's antipathy to women who lived in cities. For an odd moment, Andi was aware of an unsettling flash of…what was it?

Envy of some unknown child who might be adopted into a real family that they'd been chosen to join because they were wanted and they'd have the kind of childhood that Andi could only have dreamed about? They'd also have an amazing place to grow up in and a very cool dad who wore a cowboy hat.

Perhaps it was envy of that unknown woman who would capture Jack's heart and be with him for ever?

Or maybe it was disappointment that she belonged in such a different world and she could never be that coun-try girl, earth mother type herself? She had been a coun-try girl once. She'd lived close to here, on land that was hugged by those amazing mountains. She'd splashed in the clear water of the beautiful lakes, soaked up the summer sun and played in the snow in winter. It had been the home she had been taken away from and she would be leaving it again before long and, this time, it would be for ever.

The awareness of that impending loss only made her more aware of how much she was enjoying being with Jack and how much she was going to treasure the memo-ries of this time together.

'You may as well stay by the gate, Andi,' Jack called. 'Won't take long to get the mob down and then we can head home.'

Home…?

This part of the country might have been her home once, but the Dunlops' old house would never be *her* home. Andi was just a visitor and that was why she'd discovered the delights that a temporary freedom from necessary boundaries had been possible.

When Jack drove back down the hill, after the sheep were on their way towards the farm driveway, he had two coal black, newborn lambs on his lap, with the mother trotting anxiously beside the vehicle.

'Someone's started early,' he said. 'How cute are these twins?'

'Gorgeous,' Andi agreed. She watched the way Jack was driving with one hand and holding the lambs safely on board with his other arm and she could feel a squeeze on her heart.

Yeah…there was no denying that there were some things about being here Andi was going to miss when she was back in a big city. But there was always a price to pay for trying something different and right now it felt as if anything would be worth knowing what it was like to feel this…*happy*, that's what it was.

The soft tap on Jack's bedroom door, just before dawn, a couple of days later, dragged him out of a very pleasant dream.

Not that he'd been conscious of who the gorgeous woman he'd been kissing so very thoroughly had been, but as he pulled himself into wakefulness, he was left with an image of a tumble of long, blonde hair and a pair of rather unique, hazel green eyes.

It could only have been Andi, but it was a shock when his door opened and she was the person who poked her head around it.

'Jack? Are you awake?'

'I am now...'

'Is that you, Andi?' Dave's voice came from further down the hallway. 'Is something wrong?'

'There's a sheep right outside my bedroom window. I've been watching for a while and I can see a hoof poking out under her tail, but nothing's happening and the ewe's just walking round, lying down and then getting up again straight away. She sounds distressed.'

Jack was pulling his tee shirt over his bare chest. Luckily he'd gone to bed in a pair of boxer shorts because both Andi and his father were in the doorway now.

'Make yourself decent, lad,' Dave instructed.

Andi looked like she was trying not to make eye contact with Jack—or to give away how indecent she'd already seen him looking.

'I've got my PJs on under this oilskin,' she told Dave. 'Jack only needs to be decent enough to stay warm.'

'There's no time to waste.' Jack pulled on his jeans and the red-and-black woolly shirt.

Dave stepped back to let him through the door. 'I'd come and help, but I'm still not much use with my head in a cage.'

'We'll need some breakfast by the time we've sorted a stuck lamb, Dad. Get some more sleep if you can, but making some toast and eggs later would be more than helpful. I have a feeling we're in for a long day.'

The sheep was still in the same place. Jack could see Pingu standing on Andi's bed on the other side of the window, his small paws on the windowsill, watching them anxiously. Bess had come with them, of course, but Jack pointed to the other side of the gate.

'Stay, Bess,' he commanded. 'We don't need mum any more worried than she already is.'

Bess dropped to the ground and put her nose on her paws.

Jack pulled a surgical sleeve out of the kit he'd carried from the clinic. He was about to pull it on when he looked up. 'You should do this,' he said.

'But…'

'You know you can. It looks like one leg is tucked back, which is a common problem. She might be able to deliver on her own, but it could take a while and this is the first in a queue, so we don't want her getting too tired. Did you notice the paint splodge?'

'Oh…it's pink…' Andi's eyes widened. 'It's the triplets…'

'Put the sleeve on. I'll find some lube.' Jack reached into the kit again.

They were ready only moments later. The torch on the headband Andi was wearing was providing better light than the sun, which was only just clearing the horizon. The ground was cold, but Andi hadn't hesitated to kneel with only her thin pyjama pants between the top of her gumboots and the bottom of her waterproof coat.

This was so far from being a princess, it made Jack feel guilty for ever having thought of Andi as such. It also made a mockery of her saying that she wouldn't be good at—or enjoy—being a country vet.

She was a complete natural. And it didn't look like she was going to start complaining about the conditions she was working in or what she needed to do.

Jack held the sheep's head to keep it lying down and talked Andi through what she was doing.

'Slide your hand along the shoulder and see if you can find the foot of the leg that's turned back.'

'Yes… I've got it.'

'Keep your hand around the hoof to prevent any damage to mum and move the leg forward.'

Andi's hand reappeared. So did the second, tiny hoof of the unborn lamb. Jack could feel the ewe having another contraction.

'Good girl,' he told the sheep. 'Push hard. It should work this time.'

It did. With its nose on its forelegs like a diver, the lamb slid out fast, with the amniotic sac breaking as it landed on the ground. Almost immediately, it lifted its head and shook it, flapping the comically large ears.

'Pull it round to mum's face,' Jack directed. 'She'll be kept busy cleaning it and we can focus on the next one.'

Andi picked up the lamb. 'Oh, look at it…it's got black eyes and ears, like Pingu. It's so *cute*.'

The next baby was already arriving and it had identical colouring to the first. They waited for the third lamb with the sun climbing high enough to take the first chill off the grass. Other sheep in the paddock moved closer to see what was going on and Jack could see there were several more newborns that had arrived overnight. They were still wobbly, but they were on their feet and latching on to the supply of milk from their mothers. Jack's stomach growled and he thought wistfully of the breakfast Dave would be preparing for them.

'Could be that the ultrasound result was wrong,' he said, 'but we'd better check. I don't want to leave her to have a third lamb by herself when these two need looking after.' It was Jack who put on the long surgical glove this time. The ewe was so busy cleaning her second baby she wasn't taking any notice of what he was doing. Andi was busy, too, fitting a knitted, patchwork coat to the first arrival.

The third baby was there but Jack could only feel the tail.

'This one's small but it's breech,' he told Andi. 'I'm going to push it back into the uterus and reposition the legs. We'll need to pull it out.'

This lamb was smaller than its siblings and it had unusual colouring, being mostly black but with a white chest and a big white spot on the top of its head. It felt alarmingly limp, so Jack held it upside down and shook it gently.

'What are you doing?'

'When they come out hind legs first like that, it helps drain any fluid out of the airways.'

He put the tiny lamb on the ground then and they both watched. For a long, long moment, it lay absolutely still. Jack glanced up and he could see tears gathering in Andi's eyes, but then he saw her face light up and knew that the lamb must have at least twitched. He was aware of a warmth in his chest that was rapidly spreading right through his body. Despite being hungry and cold, Jack was feeling remarkably happy. By the time he dragged his gaze away from watching Andi's expression morphing into joy, the lamb was shaking its head with enough vigour to suggest it was going to survive but it needed help.

'This one's quite a bit smaller than the other two, so he's not going to be able to compete for a teat. We definitely need to look after him ourselves. Let's get him a bit drier and we'll try and get a first feed of colostrum into him from mum so he gets a good dose of antibodies and then we'll take him back up to the house.' Jack wrapped the lamb in an old towel and handed it to Andi. 'Looks like you've got your first one to bottle raise. Dad can look after him while we're at work, but you can have him with you in the cottage.'

Andi was beaming. 'I'm going to call him Lucky,' she said.

'Because he's alive?'

'And because he was the lucky last.' She looked down at the lamb in her arms. 'Pingu's going to love you.'

Lucky had a big cardboard box, lined with newspaper and old sacks, to sleep in and Dave would go down to the cottage during working hours, stoke the pot-bellied stove to keep the room warm and give him a bottle. After a couple of days of being on a colostrum formula, he went onto a milk replacement and he was thriving. Andi would mix the milk powder and water together, put it into a small bottle and screw the long rubber teat onto the top. Lucky would almost headbutt the bottle in his eagerness, and when he started sucking, his little tail wagged harder than Pingu's ever did and that never failed to make Andi smile.

'I love doing this,' she said. 'I'd forgotten I had a lamb to raise when I was little, but when I felt that first head bump, I could remember it. I think it actually knocked me over more than once.'

'Every country kid needs a lamb to raise.' Jack was in the cottage late in the evening after Dave had gone to bed. Bess had come with him and was in her usual spot right beside the front door—as if she was counting the minutes until she got to take Jack home again.

She was going to have to wait for a while. Jack hadn't

had any private time with Andi for a few days and he intended to make the most of this visit tonight. He wasn't going to rush anything, though, including this time before they ended up in bed. This kind of time together was special in its own way.

'You get to take your lamb to Pet's Day at school,' he added. 'And they're usually so big by then they drag you all over the rugby field when it comes time for the lamb race.'

'Did you win a prize?' Andi asked. 'With your lambs?'

'I think everybody won prizes. If it wasn't for the biggest lamb, it would be for how clean or friendly it was. I did win a prize for my sand saucer once.'

'A what?'

'It's a county school thing. You put sand in a saucer and then decorate it with flowers and leaves and twigs and stones.' Jack sighed happily. 'It was always the day we looked forward to the most. It wasn't just lambs. There were calves and ponies that could go in the dress-up competition and the grand parade at the end, which usually turned into complete chaos. There was a rabbit that escaped once, never to be seen again, and Barry Wrigley's cat ate Jendi's pet mouse when she accidently dropped it. She cried for a week.'

'I'm not surprised. Poor Jendi…' But Andi was laughing. 'Were there guinea pigs? Please tell me there were guinea pigs.'

She was teasing him, but they were both remembering how scathing he'd been of her abilities as a country vet when he'd said she probably only knew how to treat overweight designer dogs and guinea pigs.

When he'd said he didn't want her here.

He'd discovered almost instantly how wrong he'd been about Andi's abilities as a vet.

It was probably just as well he'd had no idea just how much he would end up wanting her to be here. It was in moments like these that Jack realised how much he was going to miss her.

He focused on watching Lucky suck the last drops of milk out of his bottle. One day, he wanted to watch his own kids feeding orphan lambs like this. He wanted to go to school on Pet's Day and enjoy it all over again through their eyes.

He wanted…

…a family.

That was something Andi had made it clear that she would never want but, in a way, she was helping him get closer to that dream. She was showing him a big part of what was missing in his life. She'd also told him he'd better get on with finding the woman who was going to be the mother of all those kids he wanted to fill the homestead with.

She was right.

She had shown him something else as well.

That he was capable of trusting someone enough to risk his heart again. If things were different, it could have been with Andi, but even knowing how much he was going to miss her, the gift of knowing that he was ready to move forward was…

…well, it was priceless, that's what it was.

'You know what?' Jack had suddenly had a brilliant idea.

'What?'

'The Pet's Day at Cutler's Creek School is coming up

pretty soon. I know Dad's been asked to judge the fancy dress competition and I'm a FOCCS.'

'A fox? Don't you have to get old and grey before you can rate yourself as a silver fox?'

Jack laughed and spelt it out. 'F-O-C-C-S. A Friend of Cutler's Creek School. Most people in town are. It means we're all part of fundraising for the school. There'll be a group running the BBQ as a fundraiser and some of the kids' artworks will get auctioned off. That can get quite competitive, which is very entertaining. We could cancel an afternoon clinic and keep our fingers crossed that we don't get called to an emergency and go and check it out.'

'To see the guinea pigs?' Andi was beaming.

'Exactly…'

'Count me in,' Andi said. 'Sounds like something not to be missed.' Her declaration was finished with the loud sound of Lucky sucking on a now empty bottle. 'Time for you to go back in your box,' she told him.

But Lucky was nowhere near ready to go back into his box.

'You were right.' Jack smiled. 'Pingu does love Lucky.'

'Right now I think he's loving cleaning up the milk that Lucky's got all over his face, but the love is entirely mutual. I'm sure Lucky thinks Pingu is just a funny-shaped lamb.'

'Maybe he remembers having company in the womb. At least he's not missing his siblings. And they're certainly not missing him. We got another six new arrivals today. Lambing season will be over before we know it.'

Andi didn't want to think about lambing season being over. All going well, Dave was due to have his halo brace removed by then, and while he wouldn't be ready for any heavy work straight away, he could take up light duties and manage the consultation hours and monitoring of patients in the animal hospital and there would be no reason for Andi to stay in Cutler's Creek any longer.

The invitation to go to the Pet's Day at the school was something to look forward to, but it had a downside in that it would be another big step closer to her time here being over.

Another distraction was needed.

And Andi wanted to hear the delicious sound of Jack's laughter again. She loved that she'd made him laugh with her comment about being a silver fox. Not that he wouldn't be an extremely handsome older man, mind you. Like his dad…

Andi didn't want to think about the gap in her life that would be the shape of the two Dunlop men, either. It was time to take control.

'Watch this…' Andi went to stand near Bess by the front door. 'Away, Pingu,' she commanded, putting her right hand out to the side. 'Get away.'

Pingu obediently went right. Lucky trotted after him.

'Over,' Andi ordered, putting out her left hand. When Pingu had gone a couple of steps to the left, she added, 'Stand.'

Pingu stopped so suddenly that Lucky tripped over his own feet, fell into a kneeling position and then rolled onto the floor.

Jack was laughing. 'Look at the expression on Bess's face.'

Andi turned towards the door. It did, indeed, look as if his beloved heading dog was rolling her eyes.

She looked at Jack then and saw the crinkles at the corners of his eyes and his rumpled hair and that smile that could light up a room.

Light up a whole life, in fact.

She could feel that light as much as see it. It was surrounding her. She could breathe it in and let it settle around her heart and it felt like...love.

Pure and simple. Except it wasn't simple, was it?

This shouldn't have happened. Andi had been so sure she could protect herself from this, but she had failed rather spectacularly.

She had fallen in love with Jack Dunlop.

It was the last thing she would have allowed to happen if she'd seen it coming. The last thing Jack would have wanted to happen. She could hear an echo of his words the night they'd taken that huge step closer to each other. The night he'd offered to show her the cottage and they'd both known he hadn't been talking about her moving out of the homestead for a bit more independence.

...I mean...it's not forever, is it? You could try it just for a night or two, and if it doesn't suit, we'll never need to mention it again. Or you could enjoy it for the rest of your time here.

It wasn't forever. If she'd fallen in love, it was Andi's problem, not Jack's. Maybe she needed to take note of more of that loaded conversation. It would be best if the way she was feeling was never mentioned again. Even to herself.

CHAPTER EIGHT

THE CLOUDLESS, blue sky confirmed the perfect weather that had been forecast for the much-anticipated Pet's Day at the Cutler's Creek district school.

Excited children were outnumbered by animals and the family members who'd come to what was as much a community celebration as an opportunity for a country school to combine education and enjoyment. For many weeks now, the children had been learning about animal welfare and training as they prepared their lambs and calves and all the other family pets for their big day out.

Part of their studies about environmental issues and recycling had been making sculptures from rubbish that were now proudly displayed in one of the classrooms. A healthy food project was represented in another classroom where the traditional sand saucer competition had been upgraded to a pictorial fruit and vegetable platter.

'Look at that one...' Andi used her phone to take a photograph of a Christmas tree made of broccoli florets with a pretzel stick trunk and decorated with cherry tomato baubles, yellow capsicum lights, spaghetti tinsel and a pineapple star on the top. 'No wonder it got first prize. I'm so going to make one of these for the next Christmas function I need to take a contribution for. How good would that be with a hummus dip beside it?'

'Should go down a treat with those healthy types in Auckland.' Jack grinned at her. 'You could make one for your personal trainer.'

Andi shook her head. She wasn't going to take the bait.

Jack didn't seem bothered. 'Are you and Pingu happy to wander about for a bit longer?' he asked. 'There's a couple of people I need to catch up with. How 'bout we meet by the BBQ in half an hour or so? You don't want to miss one of Pete's famous bacon-and-egg bread rolls.'

'I'm happy,' Andi told him. She was way more than happy, if she was honest. Spending time like this, with Jack, that had nothing to do with work was like a free pass to think of him as something other than a colleague.

As a friend.

As a lover.

And, okay…it wasn't a good thing that she had fallen in love with him, but there was nothing she could do about that now and it wasn't proving too difficult to keep under control. She had, in fact, been more successful than she could have imagined in keeping it entirely to herself. Andi knew there would be a price to pay down the track because, as Jack had set out in the terms of engagement, it was only to be enjoyed during the time she was here and there was no denying that Andi was enjoying it. Very much, indeed.

It was delicious. Addictive. Andi had never felt the drug-like euphoria of falling in love and it was obviously impossible to try and simply switch it off. Why would she want to, anyway? If she was going to have to pay for it later, she might as well make the most of it now.

She smiled up at Jack. 'Pingu and I might go and see if there are any guinea pigs next.'

'I think the small pets are behind the chickens and ducks. Over near the bike sheds. Come outside with me and I'll point you in the right direction.'

As soon as they stepped out of the classroom block, two small children came running towards them.

'Uncle Jack... Uncle *Jack*...'

'Hey, Milly...' Jack crouched to hold out his arms. 'And Hugo...how's my man?'

The children hurled themselves into his arms, but then Milly spotted Pingu. 'Oh, he's so *cute*. Can I pat him?'

'Of course you can.'

'Good girl for asking,' Jack said approvingly. 'Some dogs are scared of strangers and they might bite.'

The parents weren't far behind these children.

'Hey, Jack...'

He quickly introduced Andi. 'This is my mate Zac and his wife, Liv. They're both doctors at the local hospital. That's Milly, who goes to school here, and this is Hugo.' He hoisted the small boy onto his hip and looked across at Liv. 'I can't believe how big he's getting. Hard to believe he was such a premmie not that long ago.'

'He was premature?'

'Twenty-nine weeks.' Liv nodded. 'He was in NICU in Dunedin for a long time.'

'That must have been tough.'

'It was,' Zac agreed. 'But, on the bright side, we ended up getting JJ here as a locum and she's still here. She got together with Ben, who's the senior paramedic at our ambulance station. Love at first sight, it was.'

Jack was laughing. 'I think there was a bit more to it than that.'

Country people, Andi thought as she listened to the warmth in their voices. They were all part of each other's lives. For a city dweller like herself, it felt like it could be unwelcome and intrusive, but there was another side to that coin, wasn't there? The support that was there when you needed it. The shared memories that strengthened bonds and made even a tiny moment, like mentioning Hugo's successful fight for life as a newborn, something to celebrate again.

Liv reached up to ruffle Hugo's hair. 'You're a big boy now, aren't you, darling?' She shook her head. 'I have no idea how time just evaporates like that. Hugo will be starting school soon and we'll have to raise two lambs for Pet's Day.'

'I see our daughter has fallen in love with your dog,' Zac said to Andi. 'Can't say I blame her. What breed is it?'

Andi's gaze flicked across to meet Jack's and there was a frisson of a different kind of shared memory. One that was just between the two of them and came with the tightening of an invisible bond.

It was Jack who answered. 'He's a schnoodle.'

'Sounds like a German snack food.' Zac laughed.

'His name's Pingu,' Andi said.

'Like the penguin.' Milly sounded delighted. 'Mummy, can we get a dog just like Pingu?'

'We'll talk about that later.' It sounded like a practised parental response. 'We need to go and see Chops and get ready for the lamb race now.'

Chops? What was it with the way people named their pets around here? Andi shot another glance at Jack, but he just grinned at her with a quirk of an eyebrow that suggested it could be a case of the pot calling the kettle black.

'Ben's here,' Zac told Jack. 'He's doing the first aid cover for today. Someone in Milly's class has already fallen off her pony.'

'That was Chloe,' Milly said. 'Mummy, can I get a pony?'

'We'll talk about that later, darling. You know a pony needs more space than our back lawn. Come on, kidlets...' She reached for Hugo, but he wrapped his arms tightly around Jack's neck and hung on.

Jack just laughed. 'It's okay. I'm going in that direction, anyway, to find my dad.' He pointed towards a long, low building. 'Those are the bike sheds,' he told Andi. 'See you soon, yeah?'

He took his hat off and put it on Hugo, who looked as though he'd just been crowned as he gazed up at Jack adoringly, and Andi felt a sudden squeeze in her chest. She remembered telling Jack that he needed to get on with having that tribe of children. It had been very clear that he wanted to be a father. He had a heart big enough to consider adoption, even. What hadn't been clear, until now, was just how good he would be at it. He genuinely loved kids, didn't he? He was a natural.

She watched as the black cowboy hat disappeared into the crowd of people. Jack Dunlop was a man who loved animals and kids. A man who was kind and smart and enough of a rebel to be so astonishingly attractive. He could have any woman he wanted, if he put himself out there. How sad would it be if he'd been so badly burned that he was now at risk of missing out completely?

Andi took Pingu towards the sheds and found they

had been emptied of bikes in order to make space for crates containing an impressive variety of poultry, with hens and some tiny chicks, ducks and even a goose that hissed when it saw Pingu. There were rabbits in here as well and even a pet rat, but there were no guinea pigs to be seen. After admiring all the animals and reading the stories attached to the crates that children had written and illustrated about their pets, Andi headed off to find the BBQ, but Jack hadn't arrived at their meeting point yet.

She did see someone she recognised, however.

'Glenys…hi! How's Marigold doing?'

'So well. We've got her calf here today. My youngest son, Alfie, has been putting in the hours to train it to walk on a lead so they can go in the grand parade. He's *so* excited. Oh…' Glenys turned to the older woman beside her. 'This is my mum, Shona Bailey. Mum, this is Andi. She's the locum vet who's been here helping while Dave Dunlop is out of action.'

Andi held out her hand. 'Pleased to meet you, Shona. I'm Andi. Andi Chamberlain.'

'Chamberlain?' Shona blinked. 'That's a name I haven't heard in too many years. My best friend in high school, Sarah, became a Chamberlain when she got married.'

'That was your friend that died in that horrible car accident, down by the bridge, wasn't it?' Glenys gave her mother a sympathetic glance.

'Yes…' Shona was staring at Andi. 'She had a little girl,' she said softly. 'Andrea…'

Andi was staring back at Shona. She didn't have to say anything.

'Oh, love…' Shona wrapped her arms around Andi. 'I

never got the chance to tell you how sorry I was. I think about your mum every day. She was such a lovely woman...'

Andi was blinking back tears.

It was the spontaneous hug, as if a stranger genuinely cared about her.

It was the sudden connection to her mother—the person who'd been the centre of her world but was now more of an emotion than a real memory.

It was the feeling of...belonging?

As if she had turned a corner and she was on her way home...

Shona was still talking quietly.

'I never thought I'd see you again, love. By the time we heard about the accident, you were gone.' It sounded like Shona was welling up, too. 'I mean, it was fair enough that your grandmother came and whisked you away, but... we were shocked that she didn't bring you back for the funeral.'

Andi pulled back from the hug. 'There was a funeral?' She swallowed hard. 'I was only told my parents were cremated and their ashes scattered somewhere in the mountains. That there was no grave that I'd ever be able to visit.'

'That's true.' Shona nodded. 'But there was a huge funeral. People came from all over Central Otago. Your dad was one of the best ski guides around and your mum was an amazing nurse. You need to know how much they were loved. And missed. How much *you* were missed. I'll never forget the day we went to put the cross up. I used to go every year, on your mum's birthday, and put some flowers there but...' Shona bit her lip. 'I haven't been for a long time now. It may not even be there any longer.'

'It's still there.' Blinking wasn't doing the job any longer. Andi had to brush tears off her cheeks. 'I've seen it.'

Shona put her hand on Andi's arm. 'Get my address from the Dunlops—they know where I live. Come anytime and I'll have the kettle on. I can tell you so much about your parents, if it wouldn't be too hard for you. I've got photos, too.'

Glenys was glancing at her watch. 'Sorry, Mum, but we'd better go. Alfie would be very upset if we miss the fancy dress competition. Are you coming, Andi?'

'In a minute.' Andi needed a quiet moment to herself. Such strong emotions were buffeting her she was in danger of losing her footing and being in a crowd might be too much.

Visiting Shona to look at old photos and talk about the family she could have had and the community she could have lived in would definitely be overwhelming right now.

And...dangerous? Did she want to see and hear things that would bring back long-buried memories? It wasn't that long ago that she would avoid any mention of just this geographical region. Deliberately seeking out information on the people she'd lost would be guaranteed to open old wounds, wouldn't it?

Andi picked Pingu up to give him a cuddle as she walked to the periphery of the colourful, noisy scene with an atmosphere like nothing she had ever experienced on school grounds, but Pingu wasn't happy at being taken away from all the attention and excitement of the rural circus of Pet's Day. He wriggled to be free and on the ground again.

She put him down but stayed where she was, taking a

very deep breath as she tried to make sense of something she'd never allowed herself to feel before.

Because the overriding emotion that Andi was left with as Shona and Glenys walked away was one of a bone-deep yearning for that family she'd lost. For the kind of community that she'd been taken away from. The kind that a place like Cutler's Creek could provide.

And it was a yearning to try and find it again instead of locking it away as something to not even think about. Andi was yearning to have her *own* family. A life partner. *Children...?*

Dear Lord, where had *that* come from? The thought was so far away from the future she'd envisioned for herself and so far out of her comfort zone that Andi felt a shiver run down her spine.

Pure fear...

A fear that had been born when she'd been trapped in the back of that car so many, many years ago and she had known, on some level, that her world had ended. It was a fear of loss that had never entirely gone away.

She could see prizes being given out in the fancy dress competition to the sound of clapping and cheering. She could see a very fat lamb wearing a tutu and another one that was dressed as a Christmas elf. She spotted Marigold's calf, who was dressed as a rugby player with a striped shirt and shorts on. A red rosette was attached to his halter now and, even from this distance, Andi could see the wide grin on Shona's grandson's face.

She could see something else as well. A figure that was coming towards her from the crowd of people admiring all the pets in fancy dress.

Jack.

He had something in each hand and a smile on his face that somehow doused almost every flicker of that fear Andi had been grappling with.

'One of each,' Jack said. 'In this hand, I have sausage wrapped in lovely, unhealthy white bread with onions and *both* mustard and tomato sauce. In this hand, I have a posh Italian bread roll that is stuffed with crispy bacon and a fried egg. There's a bit of mustard and sauce in there, too. You get to choose which one you prefer.'

'Oh...' Andi was basking in the feeling of that fear ebbing. It felt like...safety? 'I'm not sure I can choose between those options,' she said, her tone very serious. 'They both sound perfect.'

'I have a solution.' Jack was still smiling. 'Let's share them. Half of each. The best of both worlds.'

They sat on the grass and ate their lunch and every bite was delicious.

If only life could be sorted so easily, Andi thought. If it was possible to share things as different as living in the city versus the country and make it work. Or if it was possible to move on from trauma in the past and not let it control what sort of future you could dream of?

'Come on...' Jack got to his feet and held out his hand. 'It's going to be time for the grand parade soon and you don't want to miss any of that.'

Andi let him pull her up. He was right, she didn't want to miss any of it.

And maybe there were other things she didn't want to miss. It was too big to even think about just yet, but...was it possible that she could choose a completely different future than she'd been so determined to provide for herself?

She'd come to Cutler's Creek believing that she belonged in Auckland and that was where she wanted to be for the rest of her life. That she would never, ever want to have children of her own.

But Shona had made her realise that far more of her than she would have believed belonged *here*, in Central Otago.

Where Jack would always belong.

Was it possible that Andi could belong with him? That *she* could be the mother of the children he would be such a fabulous father for?

No…the idea was big enough to be fanning a spark of that fear and Andi didn't want to spoil memories of a day she knew she was going to treasure for the rest of her life.

Like every day with Jack?

'Come on, Pingu,' she said brightly. 'You have no idea how exciting this grand parade is going to be.'

It was Bess who woke Jack in the middle of the night after the Cutler's Creek School's Pet's Day, with a nudge from a cold, damp nose.

He lay there for a minute in the dark before he heard the sound, but Bess was already waiting by the door as he leapt out of bed moments later.

Jack went straight to the laundry, where the whelping box filled the space between the washing machine and the old concrete tubs.

'What is it, Meg?' He ran his hands over the dog who was panting and shivering and clearly in distress. Jack could feel the next contraction as it started, but there was no sign of a puppy arriving. 'How long have you been like this, girl?'

He offered Meg some water, but she didn't drink any.

He watched her for another ten minutes but then went and pulled his clothes on and tapped on his father's door.

'Meg's in labour,' he told Dave. 'And I think she might be in trouble. I'm going to take her over to the clinic and do an ultrasound.'

'I'll come with you.' Dave was quite practised in getting himself in and out of bed with the brace on now. 'Throw me a shirt, lad. And a jumper. It'll be a bit chilly out there.'

Thirty minutes later Dave was making a phone call. Jack went, with Bess at his heels, to the shearer's cottage to knock on the door and then open it. He reassured a barking Pingu, looked at Lucky, who was trying to climb out of the pen he now had in the corner of the living room, and then felt a wash of relief as a tousled but alert Andi appeared at her bedroom door. She was wearing the leggings and oversized tee shirt that were her pyjamas.

'What's happened, Jack?'

'It's Meg. She's in labour and she's got a pup stuck in the birth canal. The other pups are getting distressed, so we'll have to do a Caesarean if we're going to save any of them. We need all hands on deck. Dad's ringing Maureen, so she should be here in a few minutes, but…but I need *you*, Andi.'

He did. It wasn't just for her medical skills, although he wanted the best for his dog and her babies. He needed Andi in more than a professional role. She knew him— probably better than any other woman had ever known him. She understood how important this was to him and… well…he just needed her by his side, it was as simple as that. Could Andi see that, in his eyes, as she held his gaze?

She seemed to. She certainly didn't waste a moment,

not bothering to go back for clothes, just throwing on the oilskin coat hanging on the wall beside the front door.

'Let's go,' she said quietly. 'Pingu—you stay here this time. You can keep Lucky company.'

'You better stay here, too, Bess.'

Bess didn't look at all happy at being left behind and Jack wasn't sure why he shut her into the cottage with Pingu. Maybe he didn't want anything to come between himself and Andi right now as they faced a challenge that could well turn into a catastrophe. He wanted to feel that bond. To lean into the strength it was capable of providing.

'I don't know how long she'd been in labour before I found her, but it could have been a while. She'll be dehydrated.'

'We'll set up IV fluids and electrolytes as a first step, then.' Andi nodded. 'Do you want to do the anaesthetic?'

'Yes. I'll give her a general but combine it with an epidural to cut the amount of drugs she'll need. That'll help the pups as well as let her wake up in better condition. Are you happy doing the surgery?'

'Want to know a secret?'

He did. He wanted to know what could make her look at him with that kind of glow that made him feel so much happier. Hopeful. More confident, even, as though they could cope with anything as long as they could do it together.

'Tell me...'

Andi smiled at Jack. 'C-sections are my favourite surgeries.'

Maureen was driving up to the animal hospital as they arrived. Dave was already inside, setting Theatre up with everything they needed for the surgery and resuscitation of the puppies. Andi scrubbed in and was gowned, gloved and masked by the time Jack had administered the anaesthetic and Maureen helped him position Meg on her back, shave and disinfect her abdomen. The tension ramped up as Andi took her position and picked up a scalpel.

Jack looked up as he adjusted the volume on the heart rate monitor, as if he felt the glance Andi was giving him before making that first incision. Between the elastic of her hair cover and the top of the mask pinched in at the bridge of her nose, he could see her eyes. He'd never seen anyone else with that unusual green shade of hazel. He'd never felt anyone else imparting this kind of reassurance, either.

It's okay, Jack. I've got this. We've got this...

Her incision was confident. She brought the uterus into view at the top and then very carefully and precisely opened it with a pair of scissors.

'I'll take the stuck pup out first,' she said.

Jack watched the movements of her hands as she extracted the puppy in what would probably be the most difficult part of this surgery. Maureen was waiting with a towel to take the pup which, as expected, was completely limp.

Everything seemed to speed up after that. Puppies and placentas were gently lifted out of the uterus, the amniotic sacs removed and the pups given to Dave, Maureen and Jack as he stepped back to help while still monitoring Meg. The puppies needed to be rubbed and dried and given some oxygen. The squeaky, first cry of the one Jack was working on almost brought tears to his eyes.

Six puppies in all. Only the one that had been stuck

hadn't survived. They were all in a basket under a heat lamp by the time Andi had stitched up Meg's uterus and closed the abdominal incision and Jack reversed the anaesthetic and carried Meg to a warm, comfortable crate to wake up properly.

Maureen whisked instruments into the washer disinfector, dealt with contaminated linen and then bustled Dave out to take him back to the homestead.

'It's the closest you've been to working again for weeks and…the stress! Goodness me, I need a bit of a lie-down myself.' She took one more peek into the basket of puppies. 'They're gorgeous. I think I want one myself.'

'You don't need a huntaway, Reenie.' But Dave was smiling. 'Might be time I got a new pup, though.' He crooked his arm. 'Come on. Let's go and put the kettle on and I'll make you a nice cup of tea and we'll talk about which puppy I should pick.'

Jack watched the way Maureen slipped her hand around Dave's arm. She even laid her head against his shoulder as they vanished through the door. It wasn't the first time that Jack had wondered why his father hadn't taken their friendship any further. Were the ghosts of his first marriage still haunting him enough to prevent him from moving forward?

Jack wasn't going to let that happen to himself. He knew the future he wanted and it had a loving partner and a bunch of kids in it.

And lambs and ponies and…puppies.

He went to the basket and looked down at the tiny, sleepy babies. A couple looked like their mother, but the others were mini Jeds. Jack was gently scooping one of them into his hands as Andi came over to join him. He held it up, close to his face.

'Are you going to be as scruffy as your dad? I hope so...'

'I'm sure he's going to end up being a champion.' Andi reached out and touched the puppy's head with her forefinger. 'How could he not with the parents he's got?'

Jack held her gaze. 'Thank you,' he said softly. 'We might not have any of these babies if I hadn't had you to help. I'm so happy you were here.'

Andi looked a bit embarrassed by the praise. She reached into the basket to pick up another one of the puppies. 'I came to tell you that Meg is waking up. Shall we introduce her to her babies and see if she's ready to feed them?'

They carried the puppies over to where Meg was lying on her comfortable blanket. Andi crouched and held out the pup for Meg to sniff.

'This is your baby, you clever girl,' she said. 'She looks just like her mama, doesn't she?'

Having sniffed the puppy and given it a lick, Meg lay down on her side and closed her eyes again. Andi held the puppy to her abdomen and put its mouth against a teat. When she squeezed a drop of milk out, the puppy opened her mouth and latched on. Andi put her down carefully and they waited a minute to make sure that Meg wasn't distressed by what was happening.

Then, one by one, they introduced her to her other babies and helped them latch on. Andi paused with the last puppy in her hands. She held it for a moment, tucked under her chin, and she looked up at Jack, her eyes shining with what could only be happy tears. 'They're *so* adorable...'

Jack's smile felt poignant. He watched Andi crouch to settle the last puppy amongst its happily suckling siblings. How could anyone who so clearly adored babies be so sure they never wanted kids who didn't have four legs?

It was kind of sad because he was quite sure that Andi would be a wonderful mother. He could so see her holding a baby in her arms rather than a puppy.

His baby...? *Their* baby?

As Andi got to her feet, without either of them seeming to initiate it Jack found her in his arms. Just a hug, but it was suffused with the joy of new life and the satisfaction of helping a happy ending to happen. He bent his head and pressed his lips to Andi's hair. She'd discarded her theatre cap along with the other surgical clothing and her hair was still as tousled as it had been when he'd dragged her from her bed earlier tonight.

It tickled his lips and teased his nose with the scent of...

...of Andi, that's what it was.

He breathed it in. Slowly. Deeply. He could feel her against his body, and when he tightened his hold a little, getting ready to let her go, he could feel her heart beating against his skin.

And that was when he knew what had been there, hiding in plain sight.

He was in love with Andrea Chamberlain.

He wanted her in his life.

He wanted *her* to be the mother of his children.

Oh, *help*... Jack let Andi go, hoping against hope that she hadn't absorbed any of those lightning-fast thoughts that had just streamed through his head—and his heart.

She'd run for the hills if she had.

Jack felt a bit shaken himself, to be honest.

Maybe it was just a combination of the lack of sleep and the drama of the emergency surgery. It would definitely be better to pretend his thoughts had never strayed into such unacceptable territory because it would change… everything.

'Why don't you go and try and get a couple of hours' sleep?' Jack was relieved by how normal his voice sounded. 'I'll stay here and keep an eye on Meg and the babies and top up her pain relief if she needs it.'

Andi wasn't quite meeting his gaze—as if she had been aware of something that was disturbing in that hug. 'That might be a good idea…' She turned away. 'Thanks, Jack.'

CHAPTER NINE

MAYBE IT *WASN'T* such an impossible idea.

The alarm bells that had been such a strident warning on the night Meg's puppies had been born gradually wore off over the busy days that followed.

By the time the puppies' eyes and ears were opening nearly two weeks later, Jack was not only over the shock of realising that he was in love with Andi, he was starting to believe that it could actually work.

He was in the kitchen in the old homestead, opening a bottle of what had become a favourite wine to go with a platter of olives and cheese in the time before dinner, when it was now a firmly embedded routine of joining Dave out on the terrace to wind down after a full-on day in the animal hospital and heading all over the district for farm visits. It was even more enjoyable these days because they got to spend time with Meg and all her babies.

Jack hadn't said anything to Andi about how he felt, of course. He was only just getting his own head around it. He would have to say something, otherwise time would run out and she'd disappear back to Auckland but, for the moment, he was happy to simply enjoy being with her and collect even more clues that might give him more confidence to completely smash what had been an impen-

etrable barrier in choosing a life partner ever since his
marriage had ended.

Not that he was going to compare Andi to Roz because
they were completely different. The truth was that Andi
wasn't a born-and-bred city girl. She had not only spent
her most formative years in the country, she'd lived pretty
much just down the road from Cutler's Creek. She might
not remember it, but this land and the kind of lifestyle
that went with it were a part of her DNA. And yes, she'd
been adamant when she arrived that the city was her home
and where she belonged and wanted to stay for the rest of
her life, but Jack was becoming less and less convinced.

She was *happy* here.

Andi clearly loved being in charge of clinics in the
animal hospital, doing surgeries and then caring for the
inpatients afterwards, but she was more than willing—
and capable—of the big animal challenges that were the
backbone of a rural veterinary practice and often needed
the skills of two vets.

Jack was quite sure it wasn't just work that she was enjoying. She might well be missing the kind of social life
she had in a big city, but he was willing to bet that she'd
forgotten she ever used to wear white jeans and shoes with
heels on them. She was in her overalls and gumboots for
a good part of every day now. She hadn't even started
that flash red car of hers in weeks. When she'd gone into
the township a few days ago, to buy some shampoo and
grooming tools to try and do something about Pingu's
overgrown and tangled coat, and he'd asked her to pick
up some more supplies of lamb milk powder at the farm
shop, she'd borrowed one of the Dunlops' utes.

'Always wanted to try driving one of these boys' toys,'

she'd said with a grin. 'And I wouldn't be able to fit sacks of milk powder in my car.'

She was going through quite a bit of that milk powder herself, feeding Lucky, who had grown faster than his siblings who had stayed with their mother. He slept outside in one of the shearing shed pens now and went out into the paddock during the day to join the large nursery of lambs. Jack would often see Andi hanging over the gate at lunchtime or after work when she'd finished feeding Lucky, a huge smile on her face as she watched the antics of the lambs running around and leaping into the air.

Pingu was missing his best friend and it had been Jack's idea to use Bess to help further his education in becoming a sheepdog when he saw Pingu and Lucky playing outside Andi's cottage. It might not have worked, because Lucky just wanted to play with both the dogs, but man, it had been funny. The look on Bess's face when both Pingu and Lucky had been trying to herd *her* had been priceless. The look on Andi's face when she was laughing and her eyes were sparkling was just as memorable.

The look on her face much later that night as she snuggled into his arms had actually brought a lump to Jack's throat. Or had that been because of the most astonishing sex Jack had ever experienced? Who knew that sex could be so passionate but heartbreakingly tender at the same time?

He couldn't remember it ever being like this before. Not with anyone, even the woman he'd loved enough to marry. Why was this so different? Had he never discovered just how deeply it was possible to fall for someone?

Was it because he was truly making love for the first time in his life and not simply having sex…?

Phew… Jack had to shake off the memories of last night before he went back outside. He couldn't believe that he and Andi had managed to keep their private time a secret for so long, but Dave didn't seem to have a clue and Jack wasn't going to say anything about that, either.

He didn't want to put any spokes in a wheel that might be rapidly reaching its destination, but it was still running so smoothly it seemed a shame to risk it crashing to a halt before it had to.

Not that Andi had said anything recently about any plans to head back to Auckland in a hurry. Or about that partnership she wanted so badly that it was the reason she'd agreed to come to Cutler's Creek in the first place.

Jack carried the platter and wine out to the terrace. He could see the playpen that had been set up out there to let the puppies have some outside playtime and give Meg, who was snoozing on a blanket beside the pen, a break from the constant demands for food and attention. The puppies were all bumbling around, tiny tails stuck straight up in the air and miniature paws being used to poke their siblings. One puppy was gnawing on another's ear, but Andi and Dave didn't seem to be watching the antics. As Jack walked towards the table to put the platter down, he saw Andi awkwardly hugging Dave around the ironwork of his brace.

She beamed at Jack. 'It's such good news, isn't it?'

'What's that?'

'That Dave's getting his halo brace off next week.' She turned back to Dave. 'How do they do it? With sedation or local anaesthetic?'

'No. Apparently it's not that painful. They loosen the nuts on the vest and remove the upright rods and they just use a screwdriver to loosen the pins and get them out. Zac could have done it here at Cutler's Creek hospital, but I need to see the team in Dunedin for X-rays and the physio for a new set of exercises, so I'll get it done while I'm there.'

'Have you got someone to drive you? I could do it— I've never been to Dunedin.'

Jack laughed. 'You'd have to take Pingu and Lucky or you might look in the rearview mirror and see them chasing you down the highway.'

Andi shook her head at his nonsense, but she was smiling as she turned back to Dave. 'You'll have a wobbly neck for a while, won't you?'

'I think I get another sort of cervical collar to wear until I can strengthen my muscles again, but it'll still feel like total freedom, I expect.'

'I'm sure it will.' Andi's tone was soft. 'I'm so happy for you, Dave.'

She genuinely was, Jack thought as he handed her a glass of wine. He added that to the bank of evidence he was collecting that she belonged in Cutler's Creek.

Andi was already part of the family, wasn't she?

Dave looked misty enough to suggest he was thinking along the same lines. 'You're a sweetheart,' he said. He touched his glass to hers. 'We're going to miss you so much when you've gone back to the big smoke. I hope you'll come and visit again.'

For a heartbeat, Andi looked as though leaving Cutler's Creek was the last thing she wanted to do.

Jack tucked that impression away as well.

'I hope so, too,' she said. 'Don't tell Warren, but you're a way better father figure than he's been. Which has just reminded me of something I want to do before I go.' She reached into a back pocket of the faded blue jeans she was wearing and took out a small object. 'I found this in the gift shop when I went into town the other day.' She put it on the table beside the platter.

It was a small heart shape that was painted with tiny blue flowers.

Andi must have seen his slightly puzzled frown.

'They're forget-me-nots,' she told him. 'I want to attach it to the cross that's still by the bridge where my parents died.'

There was a moment's silence that was broken by Andi. It sounded as if she was making an effort to keep her tone cheerful. 'I'm just wondering what the best way to attach it would be. Can I borrow a hammer? And ask for a nail?'

'What's it made of?'

'It's ceramic but it's got a hole at the top, so it could be worn as a necklace. I thought it could hang on a nail.'

Dave was shaking his head. 'It could get knocked off. Or stolen. I think Liquid Nails would be better to glue it on securely. I've got a tube of it in the workshop. I'll find it tomorrow.'

'Thank you.' Andi picked up the heart and put it back in her pocket. 'You'll need to tell me how to use it. I've never been big on DIY.'

'I could come with you,' Jack offered. 'We could take the horses. There's a lovely cross-country ride over to the river and then following it back to the road. We could finish work a bit early for once and take some time to enjoy this lovely weather we're getting.'

'But what if there's an emergency?'

'I'll cope if there is,' Dave told them. 'Maureen can

help.' His tone was casual. 'You both deserve a bit of time off. And it'd be nice if you got to see a bit more of the countryside before you leave us behind.'

It was the most perfect late afternoon in Central Otago.

They followed tracks over the rock-studded hills and picked their way down slopes purple with flowering wild thyme that was crushed beneath the horses' hooves and released a scent that was so familiar to Andi it might have brought tears to her eyes if she'd let herself sink into the memories it stirred.

Of this land.

Of her parents.

Of picking bunches of thyme when it was in flower and presenting them to her mother. Waiting for the smile and hug she knew she would receive. The love that she would feel herself enveloped in…

Thank you so much, darling… They are my favourite flowers in the whole world…

It was unlikely that these inauspicious, tiny purple flowers could be anyone's absolute favourites, of course, but little Andi had believed it and she could still remember the pride that always came with presenting a gift she knew was going to be so appreciated.

They left the horses at the rest area, down by the river, and walked across the bridge. Andi caught her bottom lip between her teeth.

'I've never apologised properly for letting Pingu loose amongst your sheep, have I?'

'No need.' Jack's face was in shadow from the wide brim of his hat, but that only made his smile even brighter. 'If you did that, I'd have to apologise properly for all the

things I said about you being a useless townie. It's ancient history.'

So was the accident that had snatched Andi's parents
away from her. Jack helped her use the powerful glue
to stick the ceramic heart onto the centre of the small,
wooden cross. He was crouched beside her as she knelt
in front of it, but then he leaned closer and placed a soft
kiss on her hair.

'Would you like some time alone?' he asked.

'No...'

Andi scrambled to her feet so fast she lost her balance.
Jack caught her hand and got to his feet. He didn't let go
of it even when they reached the other side of the bridge
again. He didn't say anything, either, but it was obvious
her vehement response had startled him. Andi followed
him down to the river. The horses were half asleep in the
shade of a willow tree and the only sound was the water
gurgling over the rocky riverbed.

'Sorry,' Andi said.

'You don't have to apologise,' Jack said. 'I don't blame
you for not wanting to stay in a place that makes you sad.
I went years without going near where my mother's buried. It was just too hard...'

Andi took a deep breath. 'I've never told anybody this,'
she said. 'But I was in the car when that accident happened. It felt like forever before anyone came to find us
and I can remember that I couldn't undo my safety belt
and I couldn't understand why my mum and dad weren't
waking up and I was crying...'

Tears were gathering again now and they started falling when Jack folded his arms around her.

'Oh, my God,' he said quietly. 'That's horrific...'

'That's why I never, ever wanted to come back here,' Andi said. 'I wouldn't have if I hadn't wanted that partnership so much, but... I'm glad I have now. I don't have to be scared of it any longer. It's done and I never have to do it again.'

'I understand,' Jack said. 'I remember how hard it was losing my mum, but she was sick for a long time and I knew it was coming. To have that happen to you like that—and to lose *both* your parents—it's unimaginable...'

'It was only the start,' Andi said. 'My grandmother came to get me but only because there was no one else. She didn't want me. I expect she was relieved that she was wealthy enough to pack me off to boarding school as soon as arrangements could be made.'

She scrubbed at her tears with her fingers. 'I was allowed to have a pony at the school when I got older,' she said. 'And the gardener had this gorgeous old dog. A big, black one with a grey face. That was where my love for animals started. They're so good at unconditional love, aren't they? Making you feel like you're wanted...'

Jack's arms tightened around her, but Andi pulled back. She couldn't sink into what felt like love. She knew it would only make it harder to leave.

That fear was circling again. Had she really thought she could change her future and be part of a family? Not just a part but to be a *mother*? To have children and take the risk, no matter how infinitesimal that was, that they could end up with even an echo of what her own childhood had been like?

'Sadly, the best thing my grandmother ever did for me was to die,' she said quietly. 'She left me enough money to put me through vet school. To buy my gorgeous apartment with its harbour view and that totally impractical car that I've had so much fun driving.'

It felt like Jack was pulling away from her as well. Or was it that barrier between them that was expanding? Hardening into something as strong as the Liquid Nails they'd used to fasten that heart to the cross?

At least Jack knew everything about her now. Almost everything...

'That's why I could never have children,' she added. Saying the words aloud made them just as true as they'd ever been. 'You can never guarantee you'll be there to take care of them and make them feel loved and...and there's nothing worse than feeling like you're not good enough to be loved.'

The words were on the tip of Jack's tongue.

You are so much more than simply good enough. I love you, Andi...

But how could he tell her that?

That he was in love with her and wanted her to stay and...

...and have the children that she never wanted to have. To live in the place she'd never, ever even wanted to come back to.

It was a measure of just how much she wanted that partnership in the big-city practice to have faced her worst nightmare by coming back here and, having been brave enough to do that, she deserved to find the closure that she needed so that she never had to return.

It's done and I never have to do it again...

Andrea Chamberlain was the most courageous person Jack had ever met.

He loved her even more because of what he now knew about her.

And that made it impossible to say anything. Because all Jack wanted to do was to ask her to stay.

And he loved her too much to do that.

CHAPTER TEN

THE LAST LAMBS in the season were born a week after Dave Dunlop was free of his halo brace.

He was leaning on the gate of the home paddock, Jack on one side of him and Andi on the other, watching the birth that was happening in the warmth of the afternoon. Bess and Pingu were lying on the grass behind the human spectators, happy to bask in the sunshine.

None of these three skilled vets were needed to help in any way with this delivery but, like Andi, the two Dunlop men were simply enjoying the small miracle of new babies arriving in the world. The experienced ewe had broken the umbilical cords and cleared the amniotic sacs and the twin lambs had finished their head shaking and were trying to stand up, one with its legs splayed to try and keep its balance and the most recent arrival with only its back legs cooperating.

'It looks like a wee woolly wheelbarrow,' Andi said. 'I love lambs…'

'I love that it's the end of the season,' Jack said. 'No more dawn rounds or being a sheep midwife. And it's warm enough now that they won't even need coats on. Another week and we can move them back over the road so the girls can get a bit more grass.'

Andi was silent. She wouldn't be here to help with that mustering. Dave would probably be okay to start riding Mary again himself, with the new collar as some extra protection for his neck. Or maybe he'd just walk behind the mob with the dogs to help while Jack rode Custard.

In his black tee shirt and cowboy hat, like the first time she'd ever seen him.

Oh, help… Andi didn't want to think about leaving.

Leaving the farm would be a wrench all on its own.

Leaving Jack would be…

No…she couldn't start thinking about that when he was standing too close to her and might see, or feel, any hint of how overwhelmingly emotional that could be if she didn't stay in control.

She was well practised now in hiding—from both Jack *and* herself—the fact that she'd overstepped the boundaries that had been so clearly established. That this was a temporary arrangement. They both knew they weren't remotely suited as life partners and Andi could understand why Jack wasn't going to make the same mistake again by taking that kind of a risk. Why would he, when he'd been so badly hurt? Rejected, even?

Andi had tried-and-true methods to cope with the appearance of emotional storm clouds on the horizon. Sometimes a firm reminder was enough. Or physical movement to distance herself. Distraction was always good and with animals around it was usually very easy to find something to comment on.

She looked away from the newborns to the group of older lambs in a far corner of the paddock having a great game of chase and jump. Lucky was amongst them, one of the gang now. He still came running when she took a bottle of milk out to the gate, but he didn't need it. His tummy was so round he couldn't jump nearly as far as his friends.

Jack must have seen where she was looking. What he didn't realise was that he was doing exactly what she had been planning to do by distracting her. He even brought out the big guns that Andi used herself, sometimes, because they were guaranteed to succeed—the reminder of the city she would be returning to very soon.

'Want to take Lucky back to Auckland with you?' he asked, with a smile.

'I'd love to,' Andi admitted. 'I suspect the concierge of my apartment block would have something to say about it, though. Especially in about six months' time.'

'You've got a concierge?' Jack gave a silent whistle. 'You never told me that.'

Andi shrugged. 'You never asked. And it's just as well there is one, otherwise I couldn't have come down here to help out. My pot plants would have all died by now.'

Jack was grinning. 'I get it. I guess we kind of have a concierge, too. Maureen.' He tilted his head towards his father. 'When are you going to make an honest woman of her, Dad? It's obvious to everyone that you two should be together.'

Dave shook his head as he gave a huff of laughter. Then he cleared his throat and it felt like a signal that he would prefer that the subject got changed.

She wasn't wrong.

'I was saving this for when we were having wine o'clock this evening,' Dave said, 'but I can't keep it a secret any longer. I got a phone call this afternoon. From Warren.'

Andi blinked. When was the last time she'd thought about her boss in Auckland? Days ago? *Weeks...?*

'I've been talking to him, on and off, while you've been here,' Dave confessed. 'He said he was checking up on how I was doing, but we seemed to talk more about you, Andi. At the start he was just happy to hear how well you'd settled in here and how you rose to every challenge you got. He loved hearing about how well Jed's recovered after his surgery and I've been sending him photos of those gorgeous pups you saved with that Caesarean.'

'Wasn't just me,' Andi protested. 'It was all of us. You and Jack. And Maureen.'

All of us.

Telling Dave that he was a good father figure had been closer to the truth than she'd realised because this felt like the closest thing Andi had ever had to a family. She would always have such happy memories of being here.

She was even happier that the man who had the power to make or break her future had been getting such good feedback about her. It was the reason she'd come here, after all.

'I told him today that if I thought you'd be remotely interested, I'd offer you a job here.'

'What did he say to that?'

'He just laughed. He said he knows exactly where you see yourself in ten years' time—and it's not in a rural animal hospital in Central Otago.'

Andi could easily imagine Warren's words—that dismissive tone and the laughter—and she didn't like how it was making her feel. He would have been so sure of himself. So sure of what he thought Andi would be thinking and feeling. But he didn't know her, did he?

He only knew the version of her that she'd allowed the world to see.

No wonder she was so good at hiding how she felt. She'd been doing it since she was five years old and had learned that she couldn't rely on anyone else really caring about her.

Would she have to add new things to hide when she got back to the city, on top of how she felt about Jack Dunlop? Like the things that only Jack knew about her?

'I'm not sure whether I'm supposed to share this.' Dave's voice broke into her thoughts. 'But he told me they had a partners' meeting yesterday and they voted unanimously to invite you to join the partnership.'

Andi caught her breath.

At *last*…

There was a heartbeat of something that felt like triumph. Like she was holding the biggest prize ever. Andi could almost feel the mantle of respect and new status that would envelop her. This should be the happiest moment of her life so far and yet…

…it didn't feel quite right.

Andi's gaze flicked sideways to Jack.

'Congratulations,' he said quietly. 'I know what a big deal this is for you. It's what you've always wanted.'

'He sounded impatient to get you back on deck,' Dave admitted. 'Asked me more than once whether you'd booked your ferry ticket yet.'

'No.' Andi's breath came out in a small sigh as she broke the eye contact with Jack. Or had he broken it with her? 'I need to do that.'

There was a long moment's silence. Did Jack's voice sound oddly bright when he broke it?

'We'll have to celebrate that partnership this evening,' he announced. 'I'll put some of our local sparkling wine into the fridge to chill properly. It's just as good as any French champagne. I've just got a bit of urgent paperwork to do before I call it a day.'

'And I need to check on our inpatients.' Andi turned to follow him, tapping into some helpful physical distraction. 'I want to take another X-ray of that fracture I pinned this morning before I let Gizmo go home.'

The little Jack Russell terrier she'd spent half the morning operating on was a family pet but went everywhere on the farm with his owner. He'd jumped off a quad bike too soon and had been clipped by a car and it had been a challenge to save his back leg, thanks to the complicated fracture he had sustained. She needed to check that none of the bone fragments had moved out of place and look for any early signs of infection that could undo all her hard work in Theatre.

She needed to find some time to make a few phone calls or online bookings, too. The ones that would underpin her journey back to the other end of the country, but when she turned to head for the animal hospital building, she found Pingu sitting in her path, looking up at her. His black, button eyes were almost hidden by his overgrown fringe, but she could have sworn she was receiving an accusing look—as if her little dog had understood what she'd been saying about preparing to go back to their city life and it didn't stack up with the kind of adventures he now knew they could be having if they stayed in the country.

It wasn't as if she had a choice, though, was it? Even if she had, the news of that partnership made it feel as if the choice had already been made for her. She didn't have to make herself miserable by playing with any fantasies of an alternative future that was only a dream anyway.

'Look at you, Pingu.' Andi's huff of laughter felt forced, but maybe she was trying to convince herself as much as her pet. Dunking him in the river to wash off sheep dirt and cutting the knots out of his hair herself had not been a good enough way to care for her fur baby. 'I'm going to book the groomer as soon as I've sorted a ferry ticket. You weren't bred to be a farm dog, were you? You're a city dog, through and through.'

And Andi was a city girl, through and through.

That's what Jack had said himself to Marigold's owner, Glenys, wasn't it?

Had Andi used the same words deliberately?

Had she seen something in his eyes—a warning that he might ask her not to go back to Auckland and to stay here, with him, instead?

As if…

He knew how much she wanted that partnership. It represented the prize she'd worked so hard for. It would give her status amongst her colleagues and the chance to go further in her specialty. She might end up a world expert in canine orthopaedic surgery or something and travel the globe to give keynote speeches at prestigious, international conferences.

She would feel special, which was more than her grandmother had done for her. Jack's heart broke whenever he thought of little Andi as a terrified child trapped in the back of a wrecked car with her lifeless parents, but it broke even more to think of all those years of her being made to feel unwanted. Unloved.

Jack was pretty confident he hadn't revealed anything that might make Andi feel uncomfortable about leaving to go back to Auckland, however. He was, after all, an expert in hiding how he felt.

He'd had his first lessons in doing just that when he was the same age Andi had been when she was last in Cutler's Creek, when he would pretend to be happy to try and lift some of that sadness in his father's eyes that had been there ever since his mum had gotten so sick and died. He'd used the skills again during his marriage as he tried so hard to make it work, and he'd relied on them in the wake of its failure because he couldn't cope with people knowing how shattered he really was and feeling sorry for him—especially his dad.

Hiding the feelings he had for Andi was quite easy, in comparison. It was going to stop either of them getting hurt. Even a matter of minutes ago she had reinforced that what they'd found together hadn't dented her clear intention of heading back to Auckland and taking up that prestigious new partnership.

Jack emerged from the office after grappling with paperwork that was far harder to focus on than it had ever been before to find Andi still in the clinic, tidying a shelf of dog and cat worming tablets and flea treatments.

'How's Gizmo?'

'Gone home. The fracture was stable, vital signs all within a normal range and his pain relief good enough to keep him drowsy for a while.'

'Was it Murray who came to collect him?'

'Yes. I could swear he had tears in his eyes when he was carrying Gizmo out to his ute. What is it with these big, tough farmers and their dogs?'

A corner of Jack's mouth tilted upwards. 'It's just love,' he said. 'They're just better at hiding it with everything other than their dogs.'

The silence that suddenly fell felt…odd. Full of other things that were being kept hidden?

That needed to be kept hidden?

Or was it because he'd said the 'L' word? Was Andi caught by the thought of a little dog that was cared about more than she had once been?

Jack couldn't simply turn away and leave it unspoken. Not when he still had those thoughts of Andi as a terrified child at the back of his head. He wanted her to know that she hadn't deserved to be treated like that. She needed to believe that she was special. This might be the last chance Jack had to make her feel that way and he needed to do it in a way that would be memorable but wouldn't take any of the glow of what she had to look forward to back in Auckland. This was the opportunity to let them part as good friends—with no regrets.

And he thought he knew just how to do that.

'I've never taken you out to dinner.' He deliberately kept his tone as casual as possible. 'Come out with me tonight?'

'What about cover?'

'We're not on call. We are allowed to have some time to ourselves occasionally and… I'd like to take you out to dinner. As a way of saying "thank you" for everything you've done while you're here.'

Andi's eyebrows rose. She looked like she was trying not to smile. 'It was my pleasure,' she murmured.

Jack stepped closer. He leaned down to reposition a

box that had tipped on its side, deliberately letting his arm brush Andi's. His lips were very close to her ear.

'I was talking about your professional contribution,' he said, just as quietly. 'But…maybe I'd like to say "thank you" for everything else as well.'

He straightened in time to catch an unreadable glance from Andi.

'I'd love to go out to dinner,' she said. 'Give me half an hour and I'll get scrubbed up. I think I might even have a dress tucked away somewhere.'

Jack had a suit at the back of his wardrobe, and a fancy shirt that needed cufflinks that he hadn't worn since a gala ball he'd attended too many years ago to remember.

Dave's eyebrows went a lot higher than Andi's had. 'What's the occasion, lad?'

'Thought I'd take Andi out to dinner somewhere nice,' he said. He avoided meeting his father's gaze directly. 'Just to, you know, let her know how much we've appreciated having her around.'

The beat of silence made Jack look back and he caught his breath. He knew, Jack realised. Maybe he'd known all along. He knew that Jack was in love with her.

And he knew exactly why it could never work.

He'd been there when Jack's marriage had gone into its death spiral and he'd watched his son struggle to get back onto solid emotional ground in its wake. Had it been as bad for Dave as trying to help his young son come to terms with the loss of his mother? Jack could only imagine how hard it would be to watch your child suffer and not be able to fix things for them.

It was never easy for men to voice their feelings for each other, but they'd never needed to, had they?

There was a deep sympathy in the older man's eyes.

That bond was bone deep. The love infinite.

'Enjoy yourselves.' Dave smiled. 'I won't wait up.'

'Thanks, Dad,' was all Jack said. 'I'll make sure Andi has a night she'll never forget.'

Andi had been in the district for nearly three months now, but she'd never seen the waterfront in Queenstown at night.

It sparkled with light. Music drifted from bars and buskers and there were enough people to make the atmosphere on the pretty streets vibrant—as if everyone was on their way to a party.

Andi certainly looked as if she was on the way to a party. She'd found a dress in one of the bags she'd packed into her car's boot and back seat. It was badly crumpled, but after she'd hung it in the bathroom while she had a hot shower, it was almost as good as it had been when she'd worn it to a glitzy function in Auckland last year. She had no idea why she'd thought she might have any need for such a wardrobe item in a rural community but, tonight, she was very happy to put it on.

The dress was dark green. It had a solid, silk petticoat liner, but the dress was the finest see-through fabric that was decorated with tiny sequins that made it sparkle as she moved. With short sleeves, a fitted bodice and a swirly skirt, it was probably completely over-the-top for wherever Jack was planning to take her, but Andi wanted him to see her looking…well…a lot better than she had been looking for far too long, wearing her overalls and gumboots and with her hair dragged up into a messy bun. She'd brushed it until it shone tonight and simply left it loose so it tickled the skin on her back left bare by the low cut of the dress.

Judging by the look on Jack's face when she went to drop Pingu off to spend a night with Bess and Dave and Meg's puppies, she had achieved her goal. Not that Andi was basking in any admiration. She was too blown away by how Jack looked, in a suit that was almost a tuxedo. That he'd left the top buttons of his shirt undone and wasn't wearing a tie made it perfect for him. Or was the final touch even better, when he picked up his cowboy hat?

'Let's take my car,' Andi suggested. 'I'd better make sure it's running okay before I set off to drive the length of the country again. The battery might have died by now.'

It hadn't. The sleek sports car purred its way into Queenstown.

'Do you like Japanese food?' Jack queried, as they walked through a mall with fairy lights woven through the branches of tall trees on either side. 'We're heading for Beach Street and the esplanade. There's a place I've heard about that does an amazing degustation menu. Or there's a Michelin-starred restaurant not far away.'

They could see the lake now, with the lights of outdoor eateries competing with the glow from anchored yachts. Further out, the moonlight turned the water silver and lit up the silhouette of towering mountains.

Andi caught her breath.

She didn't want to be shut inside in the kind of restaurant that she could go to anytime in Auckland.

Maybe she didn't want anyone else around because she just wanted to soak in Jack Dunlop's company.

'You know what I'd really like?' she asked.

His eyes caught hers. 'Tell me…'

'Fish and chips. It's warm enough to sit outside and have a picnic. On the beach maybe?'

'The botanical gardens are lovely. Just at the end of the beach. There are places to sit and look back at the township or out to the lake and mountains.'

'Sounds perfect.'

'On one condition.'

'What's that?'

'That we don't talk about that flash job you're going back to. Or when you're leaving. Just for tonight, could we pretend that you're never going anywhere?'

The squeeze on Andi's heart was so tight she couldn't breathe for what felt like too long.

'That sounds perfect, too,' she whispered.

It was.

They bought hot, crispy beer-battered fish fillets and hand-cut chips that stayed warm long enough, wrapped in their layers of white paper, for them to find a completely private place on the beach beneath a huge willow tree. They talked about the people who were lining up to adopt Meg's puppies and that Jed was back in training for the next event on the dog trialling calendar. There was laughter to be found in remembering the day they met and joy to be shared in the relief that Dave had recovered so well from an accident that could have been a tragedy.

And then there was the kiss...

A kiss that was so sweet, so long and so tender that it broke Andi's heart.

It felt like Jack was saying goodbye.

It felt as if it might be breaking *his* heart as well, but neither of them talked about her leaving or where she was going back to, because those had been the rules for a night out that had, indeed, been perfect.

* * *

Three days later, the little red car was on the driveway again.

Pingu was clipped onto his safety belt in the front passenger seat. The back seat and boot space were once again loaded with bags—one of which included the sparkly, green dress.

Andi hugged Dave tightly and promised to keep in touch. She had to blink back tears and take a deep breath as he turned towards the house, clearly giving her a private moment to say goodbye to Jack.

But what could she say?

If she started to say anything at all, the dam holding back *everything* she wanted to say might burst and she couldn't do that to Jack.

She couldn't tell him that she loved him. Even if she could genuinely tell him that she was prepared to give up her fabulous new partnership and her life in Auckland to be with him, it wouldn't be enough, would it?

He wanted a family and she couldn't promise that she could give him the children he longed for.

Why on earth would she think Jack might want her to stay?

He'd been there and done that, with someone just like her, and it had broken him.

She loved him too much to be prepared to risk doing that to him again.

She couldn't risk her own heart, either. She couldn't bear to offer something that might very well be rejected, however kindly Jack would do that.

She couldn't bear even an echo of feeling that she wasn't loved enough. That *she* wasn't enough.

The silence between them felt like it could ignite if

someone struck a verbal match, but still, Andi couldn't find anything to say.

Jack looked like he was finding it just as difficult, but at least he broke the tension. He simply held his arms out and then they were hugging. So tightly that Andi couldn't breathe, but it didn't matter.

'Take care,' he whispered into her ear.

The dam holding back those words had become a huge lump in Andi's throat. Her voice sounded strangled.

'You, too...' was all she could say.

And then Andi was in the driver's seat of the little red car.

Driving away.

When she looked in the rearview mirror, she could see Jack standing in the middle of the driveway with Bess sitting like a sentinel by his side.

She almost put her foot on the brake so that she could stop and turn around.

Almost.

But ahead of her lay everything she'd dreamed about for what felt like all her life. Independence. Success. Security.

Behind her stood a man who would never live anywhere other than the place that held such deep-seated grief for Andi. A man who wanted nothing more than the children she could never give him.

It couldn't work. It would end up breaking both of them.

She'd known it was going to be difficult to leave. But if Jack had wanted her to stay, he would have said something, and he hadn't, had he?

'Don't look back,' she whispered aloud to herself. 'It's not the direction you're going in...'

CHAPTER ELEVEN

EARLY MORNING SURGERIES were over.

Two cats speyed, one dog neutered, a cat with an abscess that needed draining because it spent its nights fighting every other cat in the neighbourhood, and four cats and dogs who'd needed dental procedures. Designer dogs, she noted. A cavoodle and a spoodle.

She could imagine what Jack would have to say about the clientele on this morning's list. Maybe he'd say it all with simply a quirk of an eyebrow. Or a smirk. She hadn't been remotely amused by that kind of expression when he'd queried Pingu's breeding.

A schnoodle?

...should I say 'bless you'?

Strangely, it made her smile to remember it now. Jack had changed his mind about Pingu in the end, hadn't he? She could almost hear an echo of his laughter and see the crinkles at the corners of those gorgeous dark eyes when he'd watched her clever little dog following commands to try and herd Lucky around the living room in the cottage.

Andi left her patients recovering from anaesthesia in

the care of the clinic's vet nurses and rushed off to start her late morning consultations.

Warren poked his head out of his office as she went past.

'Andi…how's it going? You all settled back in?'

'Yes.' Of course she was. She'd been back in the city for three weeks now. 'Can't stop, Warren. I suspect there's a full waiting room out there.'

'I know, I know. Just wanted to remind you about the partners' dinner next week. Black tie. It's an important occasion welcoming our new partner.' He was beaming at Andi. 'Be a good excuse to treat yourself to a new dress.'

'I might just do that.' But Andi's smile felt forced. She might have to buy a new dress because she certainly wouldn't be wearing her sparkly, green one to that dinner. She might very well never wear it again, in fact, because she didn't want to tarnish the memories of the last time she'd worn it for that date with Jack, eating fish and chips on the beach under the light of the moon.

If you discounted working hours and their stolen nights together, had that been their first *real* date? Or had that been when Jack had given her a tour of Cutler's Creek on the way to cutting George the goat's hooves? When they'd started to get to know each other. When she knew their futures would be on opposite ends of any spectrum of what they wanted their lives to look like as far as a personal life and family went.

That ride up the hill to bring the pregnant sheep closer to the homestead and more feed prior to lambing had been much more like a date, though, hadn't it?

It had, after all, been the first time he'd kissed her.

A kiss like none she'd ever experienced in her life,

but that was hardly surprising when she'd never kissed a cowboy before.

But no…the night of the beach picnic had been in a very different league.

Because it was the beginning of the end.

The night of *that* kiss…

The one that held echoes of things that were being left unsaid.

If only things could have been different…

I don't want this to have to end…

Oh, *man*…as if it wasn't bad enough having thoughts of that kiss or echoes of Jack's voice lurking in the corners of her luxurious but now lonely bedroom at night, they were going to mess with her head at work as well?

She was already past Warren's door, but her boss— or was he a colleague now?—hadn't finished what he wanted to say. 'I need to remind you about that invoice, too,' he said. 'The accountant wants to process it by the end of this week.'

'I know… I'm sorry it's taking so long. I had to break a term deposit and the bank's been a bit slow.'

It was the final box to tick to sign off her partnership and the significant financial stake in the practice. To cement her future as part of the most prestigious veterinary business in the city. It should have been done well before this but, to be honest, it wasn't really the bank's fault that the process was taking so long.

Andi was finding herself curiously reluctant to take this final, ultimately binding step to confirm her commitment.

And she had no idea why.

Had she been too tired after the long trip home?

Worried about Pingu, who seemed oddly listless and off his food?

Missing the company she'd become so used to in—and out of—work hours?

Missing Jack…?

Whatever it was, it felt like the air was heavier than she remembered it being in Auckland. It took more effort to drag it into her lungs and the oxygen it provided seemed less effective in providing any renewed energy.

She called for her first patient.

'Oh, no…' She saw the signs of pain in the overweight miniature schnauzer its owner lifted onto the table in the consulting room. 'Has Gus got tummy troubles again?'

The middle-aged woman sighed. 'He's stopped eating, but he's still being sick. He won't come for a walk.'

'Have you been feeding him table scraps again?'

'He has his own biscuits on the table, but he likes my food better. What can I do? Those eyes… Look at him…' Gus's owner stooped to plant a kiss on the dog's head.

Andi bit her lip as she reached for a thermometer. What she could do was to follow the advice she'd got the last time her pet had developed pancreatitis and to stop feeding him high-fat, human food treats.

'Repeated inflammation of the pancreas can be dangerous,' she told the woman. 'It could lead to Gus developing diabetes or even liver failure.'

Her client looked contrite now. 'But you can help, can't you? That's why we come here. Everybody knows you're the best vets in town.'

'We'll need to admit Gus,' Andi said when she'd finished her examination. 'He's running a fever and he's in pain and he's very dehydrated. We'll have to put him on a drip and give him medication for the pain and the nausea. It could take a few days to get him through this.'

'I don't care what it costs.' The woman was crying now. 'He's my baby... Please...take care of him.'

Her baby... Oh, dear Lord...had Andi really thought nothing of referring to Pingu as *her* 'fur baby'? And told Jack that she'd only ever consider having the furry variety of kids and not the human kind? Because there was no guarantee that you'd always be there to take care of them and make them feel loved?

That applied to her beloved pet as much as it would to a real child and that hadn't stopped her adopting Pingu. Good grief...maybe Jack had been relieved to see the back of someone who didn't even make sense? Someone who'd been hanging out to get back to her Tai Chi and boot camps. To live in a penthouse where you couldn't even step outside and feel grass beneath your feet.

Feeling like she had something fundamentally wrong in her life didn't stop her empathy for this client and her dog, however.

'We're going to take the very best care of Gus,' she promised. 'I'll get one of the nurses to take him through to the hospital wing now. You might like to bring his own blanket in later.'

'And his toys. I'll bring his toys...'

Andi didn't say that it was highly unlikely that Gus would want to be playing with his toys anytime soon. She knew that this dog was as loved as Pingu was. The problem was that poor Gus was being killed with kindness.

Her spirits sank a little further when she found she had another overweight dog to see next. A lovely old, black Labrador with a grey face and worsening arthritis.

'It's really important that you keep up with the exercise,' she told his family. 'It helps keep the joints moving. We need to talk about his diet, too. It's going to help a lot if we can get some weight off. There are also supplements that may help.'

A panting, snoring pug with very bad breath came next. A puppy check and vaccination were a welcome change and then Andi finished up with a dog that had a bad infestation of ear mites and was continuously shaking its head. She went through to the hospital wing to see how Gus was now that he'd had some pain relief and was getting some fluids through his intravenous line.

'You've only got ten minutes left on your lunch break,' Ginny warned. 'You ran over time on your consults.'

'I know,' Andi sighed. 'But I had to clean some ears that looked like they were full of coffee grounds before I could teach the owner how to use the mite medication.' She headed for the last crate against the wall. 'I'll take Pingu out for a bathroom break.'

Pingu was lying at the back of his crate and watched Andi open the door. He used to stand there wagging his tail, ready to leap out as soon as the pin was pulled on the latch. He hadn't done that since his first day back at work here.

'Take fifteen minutes,' Ginny said. 'Twenty, even. I'll cover for you.'

There was a green space only five minutes away from the clinic, but Pingu didn't seem to be in any hurry to get there. Andi crouched on the grass beside him.

'What's up?' she asked. 'You're not running a temperature and I don't think you're in any pain. You're just not very happy, are you?'

Andi could understand that.

She wasn't exactly happy herself.

She picked Pingu up for a cuddle. He felt so different now that he'd had a makeover at the groomers. He smelt a lot nicer, too. Was that part of why he wasn't happy? Had he preferred being a scruffy farm dog?

They'd only been away from this big, vibrant city for a matter of a few months. How could it feel as if everything that had mattered had been undermined?

'It'll get better,' Andi promised. 'We just need to get used to being home again. We'll go to the beach for a walk after work, okay? You don't get beaches in the country.'

But you did get mountains and endless sky and fresh air and it wasn't at all hard to breathe.

You got to see lambs gambolling outside your window and ride a horse up the hills and do surgery on a cow called Marigold and cut a goat's hooves, instead of endless cats that needed their teeth scraped.

Andi had thought that going back to the rural spaces she'd known as a child would bring closure. That she could come back to the city she loved and never be haunted again when she was trying to avoid even thinking about that mountainous country. Instead, she was feeling torn. She wasn't avoiding thinking about Central Otago any longer. She was thinking about it far too much!

Which was why she hadn't initiated any contact with Jack yet. Or Dave. She was afraid it would only make everything harder if she opened the door to mixing these two very different worlds. It had to be better to keep a clear separation, although if Jack had contacted her, she would have responded. Probably instantly…

But he hadn't called or even texted her.

Why would he?

She was the one who'd left, after all, but it wasn't as if she had a choice. Andi had already accepted the partnership at Warren's veterinary practice—all she had left to do was to hand over her financial contribution. Auckland was the place she needed to live for her career. Possibly other major cities in the world down the track as well, for training courses and secondments to enhance her orthopaedic speciality skills. She needed to be at this end of the country for personal reasons, too. Imagine if she went back to Cutler's Creek and had to work with Jack and watch him find the right woman who would be only too happy to help him create that huge family he dreamed of because that was exactly what she wanted as well. It would be unbearable.

Andy had everything *she'd* always wanted right here, right now.

She should be happier than she'd ever been.

What on earth was wrong with her?

Jack was in his happy place.

On his horse. Out on his farm with his dogs.

'Get away, Bess,' he yelled. 'Get *away*, girl... That'll do, Meg...'

Even better, he was out with his dad again. Dave wasn't riding yet because he couldn't risk another injury this soon, but he was using the quad bike and was down by the gate, ready to open it and watch the mob of ewes and lambs flow through. The lambs were nearly as big as their mothers and it was time to separate and wean them and for the Dunlop men to start selling their surplus stock to people on the waiting list wanting to add to their own mobs of coloured sheep.

Not Lucky, though.

He didn't need to go hunting for the special lamb that Andi had bottle raised. Instead of running from Bess, Lucky was running towards her. Thanks to Pingu, he seemed to believe he was more dog than sheep. Jack fished out his phone to take a photo. That would make Andi smile if he texted it to her.

Except he knew he wasn't going to share this photo. Or any of the others he'd taken over the last few weeks.

Like the one of Marigold's incision, which had healed so well, it was invisible under the regrown hair.

He hadn't sent the video he'd taken of Jed, either, when he'd been moving without even a hint of a limp on his last check-up. Or more than one of Meg's puppies tumbling around the house in delightful playtimes in the run-up to being chosen by their new families.

There was the photo of his father and Maureen, too, on the evening they'd announced their engagement and they were sitting out on the terrace with chilled glasses of sparkling wine.

He'd send that one. Soon. When he got to the point where it didn't...*matter* so much. When he wouldn't be checking his phone every couple of minutes after he'd sent something to see if there was any response yet.

'Get in behind, Bess,' he shouted. 'Speak up, Meg... Let's get this show on the road.' He signalled Custard to take off after a pair of naughty lambs who had decided they'd make a run for it in the opposite direction. Bess was onto them as well and it was only a matter of seconds before they slotted back into the moving mob heading for the gate. The distraction had only been momentary and there he was...thinking about Andi again. Wondering what she was doing.

Hoping she was happy.

It wasn't that Jack didn't want to stay in touch with her. Far from it.

He wanted it *too* much. If she contacted him, he would be only too happy to respond, but he hadn't heard a word.

Why would he?

She was probably far too busy now that she was back in the big smoke. She had her job that she loved where she didn't have to wear overalls and gumboots and go out in the rain or wind or snow and even do surgery in a less than ideal environment. She had limitless places to go for entertainment, like movies and concerts and exciting sports events, like international yacht races on the harbour. She didn't have to hike up hills or ride a horse for some exercise—she would be looking gorgeous in some trendy activewear and doing a Pilates or spin class at her local gym. Winding down after a busy day would be far more interesting than listening to his dad's stories over a glass of wine and a few nibbles out on the terrace. Her evenings now were no doubt full of unmissable social functions. Would she be looking stunning in that amazing green dress when she was out at some highbrow event? Dancing, maybe, with the long skirt sparkling as she whirled around under the bright lights?

She wouldn't be sitting on an old, driftwood log on a beach, eating fish and chips, that was for sure.

Although...she'd looked happy doing that, hadn't she? As if she wouldn't have wanted to be anywhere else. As happy as she'd looked when she'd been riding Mary, galloping up the hill and jumping that ditch. And as for the way she'd looked after he'd kissed her on the top of that hill…

Jack's breath came out in a sigh. Roz had looked happy at first, too. Until she realised just how much she'd given up for him. What a mistake she'd made.

With the sheep through the gate and onto the road, Dave closed the gate and climbed on board the quad bike to follow the mob and take care of any sheep that thought it might be a good idea to stop and eat some grass on the way. He gave Jack a nod and a smile as he rode past. Jack could feel his father's gaze on his back and he could imagine the way Dave was probably letting his breath out in a sigh as heavy as his own had been. He'd been watching him ever since Andi had driven off that morning. He knew how hard this was, but he wasn't going to interfere. This was something Jack had to deal with alone.

Maybe that was why he was feeling so damned lonely these days…

He picked up the pace, shouting and whistling at the dogs to let them know they were running out of time. He only had another thirty minutes or so to get the sheep into the paddock beside the shearing shed to be separated later today. Jack needed to be on the road as soon as possible after that. He had a big day ahead of him with a long drive to a large, commercial deer farm and one of his least favourite jobs to do, which was to oversee the anaesthetic and pain control for the stags having their velvet removed. It was justified for both human and animal safety, quite apart from its commercial value, but it was going to be many hours of difficult, possibly dangerous and less than pleasant work and that was definitely not helping to lift his mood.

At least it wasn't something Andi would ever have to do.

Jack would need to focus hard to keep himself, the farmhands and the deer safe for as long as it took and that came with its own bonus because he couldn't afford to get ambushed by thoughts of Andi.

Of how much he was missing her.

Every hour of every day...

Dave Dunlop had a cold beer waiting for Jack when he got back from his day on the deer farm.

'Come and sit down for a minute, lad,' he said. 'I miss having a yarn at the end of the day like we always did when Andi was here.'

'You'll be having wine o'clock with Maureen soon enough, Dad. Are you still planning to move in with her after you get married?'

'It makes sense. I never intended living in this old barn this long. I wanted to hand it over to you and the next generation of Dunlops.'

'I don't think that's ever going to happen.'

'You'll find someone, Jack. You'll get that family you've always dreamed of.'

'Will I?' Jack reached down to fondle Bess's ear. 'I messed up trying to get it first time round, didn't I? Did I rush into that marriage just because I wanted that family so much? Was I so naïve I couldn't see that it was never going to work?'

'You were young. But from where I stood, it seemed like you were the only one trying to make it work, Jack.

You even moved to the city for her and we both know how much you love this land. Even that sacrifice wasn't enough.'

'I'd do it again,' Jack said quietly. 'If I thought Andi would want me to.' Because maybe it wouldn't feel like a sacrifice this time? 'If you truly love someone,' he said quietly, 'you can put what they need ahead of what you want, and it might feel like a compromise, but it shouldn't feel like a sacrifice. Maybe we could live on the edge of a city and get the best of both worlds. I'd give up the dream of having a big family if that's what it took…' His throat felt like it was closing up on him, making it hard to breathe. How could he even think of living with someone else, let alone creating a family, when it was Andi he wanted to be with?

It was Andi he was missing so hard his heart felt like it was slowly losing the blood supply it needed to survive.

'Oh, lad…' There was a catch in his father's voice. 'I know you thought I didn't know what was going on between you and Andi, but neither of you were doing much of a job of hiding it. I really thought Andi would change her mind about leaving.'

Why would she have, Jack thought, when he'd never told her how he felt?

Those words that he'd been so desperate to say to her the day he learned that the reason she never wanted to have her own children had been because she'd never felt loved after she'd lost her parents.

You are so much more than simply good enough. I love you, Andi…

Not that he'd had any idea then of how much he would be prepared to change in order to be with her. It had taken falling into the hole left behind in his life to make him realise that nothing was going to be enough without her.

'I can see how hard this is for you,' Dave said. 'I'm sorry... I wish there was something I could do to help.'

They both sat in silence for a minute.

'Maybe there is,' Jack said.

'What? Just tell me. I'll do it.'

'Look after this place and the clinic—just long enough to let me see her again. That's the only way I'm going to know for sure. We can sort out anything else after that, but I don't want to live the rest of my life not knowing.'

CHAPTER TWELVE

ANDI HAD BEEN crying right through the last appointment of her day.

So had Mrs Parker.

Sadly, the time had come for her to say goodbye to her beloved Toby, and while Andi knew it was the kindest thing to do and that she could do it without causing any distress to the little dog, it was making her own heart bleed, like it always did.

She was still wiping away tears when it was all over and she was tidying up the consulting room. Appointments like this were always scheduled for end of clinic times to prevent the grieving owner having to walk through a waiting room full of other people and their pets. Mrs Parker's son had come with her so she had all the support she needed to get through the first stage of what must feel an unbearable adjustment. What Andi needed right now was to get away from work. To take Pingu somewhere lovely, like a park or a beach, and have a long enough walk to leave the sadness behind.

'You okay?' Ginny poked her head around the door of the consulting room.

'Yeah…' Andi blew her nose on the damp handful of tissues she was clutching. 'You know…'

'I do. Um…'

Andi's heart sank. 'What's up, Ginny?'

'We've got a walk-in.' Ginny was looking uncharacteristically flustered. 'A guy with his dog. Said he's really worried about her.'

'Does the dog look sick? Or injured?'

'No. Looks like it's come straight off the farm. It's got a bit of rope for a lead, would you believe?'

'Ah…'

Andi would believe that, actually. When she and Dave had been standing on the sidelines watching Jack work with Bess in the heading dog class of the dog trials that day, Pingu had been sitting beside her in his smart matching harness and lead, but Meg had had an old piece of rope looped and tied around her collar that Dave was loosely holding the other end of.

Whoever had brought his dog into the animal hospital probably *had* come straight off a farm and that meant that Andi wasn't about to send them away. She had a totally new respect for farmers and their judgement about whether or not an animal needed professional medical care.

But why had they come here? Had a farmer come into the city for an appointment or shopping that he couldn't do out in the country and his dog had become suddenly unwell?

'Just give me a sec,' Andi told Ginny. 'And then you can bring him in.'

She blew her nose again, smoothed back any stray locks of hair and straightened her back. Being professional was exactly what she needed right now. It would remind her of the flip side of the hardest parts of this job—the times when she was needed and she could help put things right for an animal who had something wrong.

The door swung open seconds later and the dog came in first. Quite a large dog by inner-city size standards and most certainly not a designer model. This was a real farm dog, sleek and mostly black but with a white muzzle and chest and tan patches on her cheeks and eyebrows.

She looked remarkably like Bess.

It *was* Bess…wasn't it?

Andi blinked and then blinked again. *'Bess…?'* she whispered.

A tall figure was on the other end of the rope. Wearing black jeans and boots. A black tee shirt…

…a black cowboy hat…

Jack…

Andi was completely lost for words.

'Gidday,' Jack said. He took his hat off and dropped it onto the end of the stainless-steel examination table. 'I've brought my dog in.'

Andi cleared her throat. 'So I see. Ah…what seems to be the problem?'

Jack leaned down to touch his dog's head. 'I think she's depressed.'

'Oh…' Andi bit her lip, her thoughts suddenly veering towards her own dog. Pingu was definitely not feeling much joy these days. 'Is she off her food?'

'Yep.'

'Lacking enthusiasm for things she usually enjoys, like a walk, for instance?'

'Yep.' Jack was nodding. 'I reckon she's lost her zest for life. You know what I mean?'

It was Andi's turn to nod. 'I do…' She took a deep breath. 'Do you have any idea why she might be unhappy?'

'I do,' Jack said. His tone was even. Mildly surprised, almost. 'I think she's in love…but they can't be together…'

'Oh…'

Andi could feel a smile tweaking the corners of her mouth. She remembered telling Jack that she thought Pingu was totally smitten with Bess. That all he wanted to do was to sit and stare at her and copy everything she did.

But the other way around?

He had to be joking. Bess must have been more than happy when Pingu got taken away and life got back to normal. Andi hadn't forgotten the way Jack's favourite dog had growled at Pingu on her first day in Cutler's Creek— when he was beside her on the couch on the terrace, wagging his tail and desperately keen to start a game with his new friend. The way she'd ignored him in the weeks to come. That look on the face of the expert heading dog when she had to sit and watch him playing at *her* job by trying to round up a compliant Lucky the lamb.

But maybe Jack wasn't really talking about Bess at all?

Was this like that night when anyone listening might have thought he was talking about Andi moving into the shearer's cottage when he was really talking about them becoming lovers?

'Perhaps I should go and get Pingu?' she offered. 'Bess might be happier if they could spend some time together.'

But Jack sighed heavily. 'I'm not sure that just a visit would be enough. It might even make it harder. What if they see each other again but can't find a solution to the problems that are keeping them apart?'

'It might not be simple,' Andi agreed, keeping her tone

serious. 'Falling in love with the wrong person can make life very difficult.'

'It can indeed.'

'Sometimes it can be cured if you have enough time away from that person, though. To…you know…get over it.'

Andi wanted Jack to look up. So that she might be able to decide why he'd come almost the length of the country to be standing here in her consulting room.

Jack cleared his throat. 'And sometimes,' he said slowly, 'there's no cure, so you have to do something drastic.'

'Like what?'

'Oh… I dunno…' Jack finally looked up. 'Like move to the city? To be with the person you're that much in love with? Because life just isn't the same without having them around?'

It was too hard for Andi to take a breath, thanks to what she could see in Jack's eyes. It looked remarkably like a reflection of the misery that had been trying to drag her down ever since she'd arrived back in Auckland. Had she really been wondering why she wasn't feeling as happy as she should have been feeling when she'd finally achieved the biggest goals in her life? Why she'd been so reluctant to speed up the process of committing the rest of her professional life to this city and this clinic?

The reason was standing right in front of her.

The love she was feeling for Jack Dunlop in this moment was fierce enough to be threatening to melt something in her body.

Her heart, probably.

'But…' Andi would have considered herself cried out for the day after her last appointment, but she could feel new tears at the back of her eyes now. 'But Bess would hate being in the city. She'd be even more unhappy...'

'It's worth a try.' Jack let go of the rope he was holding and took a step closer to Andi. 'You've got to try something, don't you, when you don't want to live without the person you love that much...'

He was right in front of her.

He was telling her that he loved her. That she was not only good enough to be loved but that he didn't want to live without her. And he'd come all this way so that he could tell her in person? So that he could look into her eyes and see right into her soul as he did so?

'Oh, Jack...' The words were a sigh. Andi couldn't pretend they were talking about Bess and Pingu now. 'But I'm a city girl...'

'No...you're *you*,' Jack said softly. 'You're gorgeous and amazing and so, so clever and you will *be* you wherever you live and I will always love you, so if you have to be in the city to be happy, then that's where I'll learn to be happy, too.'

But Andi shook her head. 'You'd hate it.' A tear rolled from each eye as she blinked. 'I don't even like it that much now.' It was true, she realised. Everything she'd thought was so important to her in the life she'd built— like the partnership and her apartment and her car— well...they all suddenly felt...irrelevant. Far less important than how she felt about this man, who was so close to her she could feel the warmth of his body.

Jack had suddenly become very, very still. 'Why not?'

'Something's missing,' Andi said.

'What?'

'*You...*'

She saw the dawn of light in Jack's eyes. The joy. And it was the most beautiful thing she'd ever seen.

'And my heart,' Andi added quickly, because she knew Jack was about to start kissing her. 'I think I left a rather large part of my heart behind.'

She'd been right. Jack was about to start kissing her.

And what a kiss it was. Andi could feel all the heartache behind it—the unique loneliness of being away from the person you love that much. She could feel something else, too. Something beautiful.

Hope...

Jack's eyes looked misty with a mix of joy and hope when Andi finally opened her eyes again.

'I think a part of your heart has always been there. It was your first home.' Jack had gone still again. 'Do you think it could be your forever home?'

Andi was smiling through tears of happiness. 'You sound like you want to adopt me. Like a rescue dog...'

Jack was smiling, too. 'I want to marry you,' he said. 'I want us to be together for ever. But that doesn't mean you have to start having babies. I'll be just as happy with fur kids if I can have them with you.'

'Oh...' Andi could still taste an echo of Jack on her lips. It wasn't enough. She wanted more.

The idea of Jack not being the father she knew he was born to be wasn't enough, either. 'I think...' The words were tentative but only because she didn't know how Jack might react. She knew how true they were the moment they were leaving her lips. 'I might have changed my mind about having a family of my own.'

'I wouldn't ask you to do that,' Jack said softly. 'Not

when I know how you feel about it. How you'd never want to risk a child going through what you had to go through.'

'But they wouldn't.' Andi swallowed hard. 'There was nobody for me other than a grandmother who didn't want me. If we got vaporised or something, any child of ours would have a grandfather who would love them to bits.'

'A grandmother, too,' Jack said. 'Dad and Maureen are engaged now.'

'Oh… I'm so happy to hear that.' Andi was looking misty now. 'And if they ended up looking after our kids, they'd have the whole of Cutler's Creek helping them. People like Shona and Glenys and Zac and Liv and Ben and JJ and…'

Jack was laughing. 'I get it…it's a community.'

'It's the biggest insurance policy ever. One that money could never buy. It's a thread of what makes a family a family and not just a bunch of people who happen to be related to each other.'

'Like your grandmother.'

Andi's nod was sombre.

'Didn't you tell me that it's the unconditional love that makes a family a family?'

She nodded again.

'That's how I love you, Andrea Chamberlain. I'm never going to let you think that you don't deserve to be loved this much. Unconditionally. And for ever. That's how it works, isn't it?'

'Yes…and that's how I love you, too, Jack Dunlop.' Andi stood on tiptoes to bring herself closer to Jack's face. 'You're my family…'

She wanted another kiss.

No…

Andi wanted so much more than another kiss. She wanted a lifetime to love and be loved by this man.

She wanted to have his babies.

She wanted those babies to have grandparents who loved them. A community that cared. A school that could give them the joy of a Pet's Day.

Okay…she wanted it all.

And, judging by the look in Jack's eyes, he was more than happy to give it to her.

EPILOGUE

Two years later...

'YOU ALL SET, JACK?'

'I think so.' Jack checked his watch. 'We've still got ten minutes before we're on, though. You might need to get out there and be ready to release the sheep, Zac.'

'Dave's already there. He's got Tom helping him.'

Around the fenced central ring of these dog trials, spectators were already gathering. They were expecting the prize-giving ceremony to start, but they were clearly also curious about why some unusual obstacles were being carefully placed on the grass when the competition classes for both the huntaways up on the hill and the heading dogs in the ring had finished.

Dave Dunlop was off to one side of the ring, near a pair of orange road cones, beside a small pen that held three coloured sheep, one of which had a very distinctive white patch on its head.

'They know to wait until you've been introduced,' Zac said. He glanced down at Bess, who was sitting right beside Jack, and then, as everybody did, he smiled at the little dog sitting right beside Bess. Pingu was looking just as focused as his best friend. His head was tipped back so he could see the first signal that would come from his human. Still smiling, Zac lifted his own gaze.

'You sure you're okay to do this, Andi?'

'I can't wait,' she replied. 'It's our first public performance.' She caught Jack's gaze and the bond between the two of them would have been obvious to the spectators on the far side of the ring. Then Andi grinned. 'I just hope it won't be our last.'

'I was actually referring to the possibility that you could go into labour before you finish the demonstration.'

'Just as well you and Liv and JJ are here, mate.' Jack nodded. 'And Ben's got an ambulance parked out the back. I did try and suggest that Andi stay home and put her feet up, but you know how stubborn my wife can be.'

Andi looked totally unrepentant. 'I wasn't going to stay at home while the rest of my family is here.' She looked across the ring and raised her hand to wave at Liv. 'I see Grace and Milly are inseparable, as usual. Like Tom and his grandpa.'

'Those two are definitely a mutual admiration society,' Zac agreed. 'A bit like Pingu and Bess.' He shifted his gaze back to Jack.

'What's that look for?' Jack sounded surprised. 'What have I done now?'

'It's not what you've done now, mate. It's what you and Andi did when you took Tom and Grace in as foster kids.'

'Soon to be adopted,' Andi said, proudly. 'And how could we not take them in when they'd lost their mum? Grace was only five years old.'

She was sharing another glance with Jack.

Zac knew why. Andi had been that age when she'd lost her parents. When Zac had talked to Jack about the trauma of these local children losing their single mum to an aggressive cancer, it had only been a few months after Jack had come back from his journey to Auckland to try and find a way to be with the love of his life.

Dave had been engaged to Maureen by then and he had moved into her little house beside the school not long after Andi and Pingu had made their permanent move back to Cutler's Creek.

It had been Andi's idea that they foster Grace and her older brother, Tom, when she heard about their tragic circumstances.

'They need a family,' she'd said simply. *'And so do we. Besides...it'll save me having to try and get pregnant with triplets.'*

Zac hadn't asked for an explanation for what was clearly a private joke between Andi and Jack, but the whole community could feel the love that was wrapped around Grace and Tom. So much love but it still seemed like only a fraction of what was being created by the partnership between Jack and Andi.

What a joyous occasion their wedding had been that next spring, a year or so after Andi had arrived to be the locum vet after Dave's accident. There was a sea of golden daffodils around the old Cutler's Creek stone church and Grace's dress, as the flower girl, was the same colour as the sprigs of wild thyme in the bouquet that Andi was carrying.

And now their first baby was due to make his appearance and Grace had to be the most excited big sister ever. Even his own daughter, Milly, was caught up in the anticipation.

'Grace and me have decided we're sisters,' she'd told

him yesterday. *'So does that mean I'm going to be another big sister for the baby?'*

'It means you're going to be a very special extra member of the family. Like all the Dunlops are for us.'

Because friends are the relatives you get to choose, aren't they?

A squeal of feedback over the sound system had people putting their hands over their ears.

'Sorry about that, folks.' The unwelcome noise stopped and the commentator's voice took over. 'We've got something special for everyone today. You all know our local vets, Jack and Andi Dunlop, and they're here today with Jack's prize-winning heading dog, Bess, to introduce a new kind of yard challenge.' A sound that could have been a stifled chuckle came over the loudspeakers. 'This may or may not become a bold new global trend in dog trials. Without further ado… Dave? You wanna let those over-fed sheep of yours out of their pen?'

Zac knew those sheep well. Lucky, who looked like he was wearing a white hat, was the oldest. Barbie and Lulu were the lambs that Grace and Milly had bottle raised last year. They went through the open gate of the pen, but they weren't moving very far. Lucky was nosing at Tom's pockets, hoping for a treat. He gave the friendly sheep a shove in the right direction.

Bess was between the two road cones, her gaze fixed on Jack.

Pingu was right beside her, quivering with excitement.

Both Andi and Jack put their fingers in their mouth and gave a whistle that set the dogs off. Bess went to one side, her head down and body tensed, Pingu bounced in the opposite direction and the wave of laughter from the crowd was delighted.

The three sheep weren't at all fazed by this public performance. They let the dogs round them up and take them through a gate, over a little bridge and even leapt over a tiny jump made of an old tree branch. Andi and Jack whistled and shouted.

'Get away, Pingu… *Away…* Good boy!'

'Stand, Bess… *Stand…*'

'No, Lucky… Behave yourself. You don't get to be the boss.'

The crowd also shouted—between bursts of laughter and clapping.

'Go Pingu…you wee champion…'

'Go the sheep.'

The final obstacle was a hoop that was touching the ground, but Dave and Tom were holding it upright. Bess positioned herself to one side and it was Pingu who ran back and forth behind the sheep to encourage them to go through the hoop.

They all refused.

Pingu looked at Andi, who was standing beside Jack, holding his hand and laughing too hard to whistle.

'Show them how to do it, Pingu,' she called, eventually.

The little black-and-white dog went around the sheep and through the hoop. Lucky followed him instantly. Then Barbie and Lulu trotted after them and finally Bess got up and patiently walked in their wake, making it clear that she was only doing this to help her best friend.

Zac joined in the thunderous applause as Dave and Tom used treats to get the sheep willingly back in their pen and the dogs returned to get cuddles from Jack and

Andi. His smile faded as he saw the expression on Andi's face, however. Then he saw the way she looked up at her husband and the way Jack folded her so protectively into his arms and his heart melted.

He'd never seen two people more in love.

But this was no time to stand around watching. Zac knew exactly why Jack was signalling the man who'd been giving the running commentary on the Pingu and Bess show.

'Can we get a medic to the central ring?' the commentator announced. 'Ben...you out there?'

He was. So was Zac and every other available medical professional in Cutler's Creek, including this baby's grandparents.

The Dunlop family were about to welcome their newest member.

* * * * *

*If you enjoyed this story,
check out these other great reads from
Alison Roberts*

Falling for Her Forbidden Flatmate
Miracle Twins to Heal Them
Therapy Pup to Heal the Surgeon
Forbidden Nights with the Paramedic

All available now!

FORBIDDEN
FIJI NIGHTS
WITH HER RIVAL

JC HARROWAY

MILLS & BOON

To writer friends, especially the CC ladies.

CHAPTER ONE

ENTERING THE ARRIVAL hall of Fiji's Nadi Airport, Della Wilton sighed happily. Despite coming for a working holiday, the minute she'd stepped from the plane's metal staircase onto the sun-baked tarmac, her problems had dissolved, one by one.

Della hefted her overstuffed suitcase onto the airport luggage trolley, stubbing her toe in the process. She winced in pain, but not even a fractured digit could dispel her buoyant mood. Two whole weeks of sun, seminars and pro bono surgery at Pacific Health Hospital on Fiji's main island, Viti Levu. Just the boost she needed after the stagnation of the past three and a half years since her divorce.

With her cases secured, Della sought out the exit, already dreaming of snorkelling the coral reefs of the clear, pristine waters and lounging in a hammock strung between two coconut palms. She knew from previous family holidays and, more recently, her ill-fated honeymoon marking the start of her three-year marriage that there was a taxi rank outside. But she'd barely taken two steps in that direction when her laden trolley jammed to a halt, the wheels locking. Della grunted, momentarily winded from her midsection colliding with the handle bar. Trust

her to choose the duff trolley. She reversed, hoping to
free the sticky wheels, to no avail.

Another jerking halt sent her carry-on case tumbling
to the floor with a loud clatter. Della bent to retrieve it.
The back of her neck was already clammy from the heat
and humidity and the battle with her luggage. Frazzled,
she straightened. Came face-to-face with the last person
in the world she expected to see in Fiji: Harvey Ward.

'Della...' he drawled, an amused smile tugging at his
sexy mouth. He eyed her big case suspiciously, as if it
was full of sex toys, chocolate and tequila—the sad single woman's survival kit. 'Hasn't anyone ever explained
the principle of travelling light?'

Before Della could articulate a single stunned word in
reply, Harvey swooped in and pressed a kiss to her cheek.
Della gaped, disorientated, speechless and instantly and
inconveniently turned on by the foreign contact, which
zapped her nerve endings as if she'd been pleasantly elec-
trocuted. He'd never done that before. Their usual form
of greeting was a reluctant nod of acknowledgement or
a terse *hello*.

'What on Earth are *you* doing here?' she snapped,
abandoning the polite indifference she usually produced
when addressing this man—not quite a friend, although
they'd known each other for years. Not a full-blown
enemy, although, as the more experienced trauma surgeon, he *had* stolen Della's dream job in Melbourne. And
definitely not a lover; apart from that one reckless night
after the granting of her divorce order three years ago,
when, feeling rejected and embarrassed, she'd drunk too
much rosé and had temporarily lost her mind.

On cue, Della's body helpfully recalled every detail

of how it felt to be naked in his strong arms. They'd had sex one time, and she still couldn't forget.

'It's good to see you, too.' Harvey laughed with infuriating composure, by-passing Della to select a new trolley, one that appeared to have perfectly behaved wheels.

Hateful man was good at *everything.* How dare he look so cool, relaxed, and indecently arousing in his casual linen shorts and polo shirt which showed off his light tan and lean, athletic build, when Della felt decidedly in need of another shower, preferably a cold one.

'I'm here to pick you up,' he stated simply.

Della pushed her damp, frizzy hair back from her flustered face, her skin crawling with head-to-toe prickly heat. 'Oh, well, that explains everything,' she muttered, her stomach taking a disappointed dive. The last person she wanted to *bump into* on her holiday was her professional rival and personal nemesis, Harvey. Especially when he'd obviously come all the way from Australia to goad her and point out her failings, as usual.

'I heard that,' he said with an amused shrug, effortlessly transferring her suitcases from *her* wonky trolley to *his* better one. 'What…? Not pleased to see me?'

At his flippancy, Della pressed her lips together stubbornly. That was another thing that got under her skin—just like her older brother, Brody, Harvey's best friend, the man had a competitive streak a mile wide. Probably why Harvey was so at home with her family, an overachieving clan of medics. Della's parents were GPs and Brody one of Australia's top renal surgeons. As the youngest sibling, Della had grown up scared that she'd never quite make the grade, a feeling that only intensified when self-assured, arrogant Harvey had been welcomed into the family as an honorary Wilton.

With both suitcases now perfectly balanced on the re-placement trolley, Harvey shot Della a triumphant smile, commandeered the handle bar and began to stroll towards the exit, as if assured that she'd follow.

'So you're still bearing a grudge, I see,' he said, glancing over his broad shoulder, his stare brimming with the hint of challenge that never failed to raise Della's hackles.

Ever since Brody had first introduced them to Harvey— Della had been eighteen and about to leave for medical school—there'd been something about the newly quali-fied doctor, a hunger in his eyes, that had left Della mildly threatened. It was as if Harvey knew some big secret she was too stupid to see. She'd fancied him, of course, de-spite being in a relationship with her engineering student boyfriend. Harvey was a good-looking man. Even then, at twenty-three, before he'd become a surgeon, he'd pos-sessed that air of supreme confidence. But only minutes into their first conversation, it had become glaringly ob-vious that they would never get along. Their mutual con-tempt had been instantaneous, their first impressions of each other terrible.

Brody had regaled Della with the tale of some poor woman Harvey had slept with the night before but wasn't going to call again. Harvey had merely shrugged, saying, "I told her it was nothing serious". Meanwhile, Della had been upset to leave her boyfriend and do long-distance, and Harvey had joined in with Brody's teasing, throwing out an insensitive "it probably won't last". Still dreamily in love at the time, Della had taken instant umbrage to Harvey's dismissive attitude to relationships. He'd acted as if the pursuit of love and commitment was beneath him and only for fools.

'I am not bearing a grudge,' Della said, hurrying after him, although at six-two he towered over her five-foot-six, his long stride giving him an unfair advantage. 'But I should point out that you *did* actually steal my job.'

She hated the bitter whine to her voice. Of course she was bearing a grudge. Technically, the position of head of trauma surgery at Melbourne Medical Centre wasn't *her* job. Technically, Harvey had just as much right to it as Della. But having already moved from her native Melbourne to Sydney for her ex-husband a couple of years earlier, and after the humiliation of her divorce, she'd desperately needed the professional win to boost her confidence. To lose a position to Harvey, of all people, especially after she'd slept with him, had been a bitter pill to swallow, leading Della to flee *across the ditch* to New Zealand for a consultant position in order to get away from Sydney and Ethan.

'Is it my fault that they wanted the best surgeon for the job?' he said with a wink. He passed through the automatic exit doors, where a blast of conditioned air bathed Della in his sexy masculine scent.

His casual comment nudged awake her highly evolved competitive streak. 'No, but it *is* your fault that you're an arrogant control freak.' She didn't notice he'd come to a halt until she'd collided with him, her breasts brushing his arm. She looked up, her face and her body on fire. He was too close and too tall and too... Harvey.

She stepped back, ignoring the playfulness in his dark eyes, because all she could see was the intense way he'd looked at her *that* night when he'd made her sob out his name.

'Come on, Della,' he cajoled, flashing that dazzlingly confident smile as if already certain of his powers to charm, 'it's been three years since the Melbourne job. Don't you think it's time to forgive me, to bury the proverbial hatchet, preferably somewhere other than in my skull?'

'If only…' Della muttered, fuming. She reached for the trolley, yanking it away from his control. Just because he liked to be in the driving seat didn't mean he could commandeer *her*. She caught another waft of his subtle cologne, the fresh laundry scent of his clothes and the warmth of his body, and fought the uninvited and intimate memories of that one night.

Sleeping with him had served to remind her that, despite being in her mid-thirties, she'd still been an attractive woman. Who better than love 'em and leave 'em bachelor Harvey to show her a life-affirming good time free of any strings? Because when it came to sex, he'd had plenty of practice. She'd heard the stories from Brody.

'Why *are* you here?' she demanded, coming to a defiant halt. 'Not at the airport, manhandling my cases, but here in Fiji?' More importantly, why had she meekly followed him outside when she'd always done her best to steer clear? From that first disastrous meeting, they'd rarely seen eye to eye, instead bickering like a long-suffering married couple. Harvey liked nothing better than to goad both Della and every boyfriend she'd ever brought to a family event, and Della could never seem to help rolling her eyes at his latest sexploits, affronted by his attitude towards commitment on behalf of all women.

'I was invited here by Dr Tora,' he said with a casual shrug, 'head of surgery at Pacific Health. Didn't they tell you?' He took a set of car keys from his pocket and dangled them from one long, elegant and capable finger, his easy smile further fuelling her irritation.

'Tell me what?' Della's blood chilled a few degrees, despite the hot tropical air clinging to her skin. Her voice carried a whiny pleading quality that hurt her eardrums. But whenever Harvey was around, she felt wrong-footed. Unstable. On her guard. But she couldn't show any weakness.

'That like you, I'm here to run a few seminars and have offered my surgical skills pro bono.' He dropped the bombshell and sauntered towards a nearby open-top Jeep with the hospital's name emblazoned on the door.

The hairs on the back of her neck rose. Floundering, *again*, Della hurried after him with her trolley. 'What do you mean? I don't understand.' *Please let it be a mistake.* She couldn't spend her holiday with Harvey. They might actually kill each other.

'We'll be working together for a couple of weeks,' he said in confirmation, as if in no way concerned. Effortlessly, he lifted her cases into the back of the Jeep, parked the empty trolley and walked to the driver's side, pulling his sunglasses from where he'd tucked them into the neck of his shirt.

Della wobbled on her feet, disoriented and overheated as if she was spinning inside a tumble dryer. Working together? They'd never done that before. It would be a disaster. She'd have to see him every day at the hospital with no hope of avoiding his arrogant swagger or his potent sex appeal? How was *that* fair?

'You have got to be kidding me,' she muttered, a string of swear words running through her head as she yanked open the passenger door and reluctantly climbed inside the Jeep.

'I'm afraid not,' Harvey said, starting the ignition and then leaning close to add, 'Love me or hate me, you're kind of stuck with me for a while.'

Oh, how easily they slipped into their respective roles, their game of one-upmanship, even here in beautiful Fiji. But as usual, Della felt one step behind. 'No, you're stuck with *me*,' she snapped childishly, crossing her arms and staring out of the window as Harvey chuckled and pulled out of the parking space, heading for the airport exit.

Della's lovely fortnight of sun and surgery, of giving something back to her Fijian counterparts before returning to her job in New Zealand refreshed and re-invigorated, dissolved before her eyes. Oh, she'd stick it out—she'd never allow Harvey Ward, of all people, to chase her off. If he could put up with her, she would put up with him.

But two weeks working with her professional rival? Two weeks trapped on an island with a man she knew intimately? Two weeks reminded of that incredible night in his bed when she hadn't had so much as a chaste peck on the cheek since…?

It sounded more like a prison sentence than a holiday.

CHAPTER TWO

A SOLID THIRTY MINUTES. That's how long it had taken Harvey to calm down after the brief but silent car journey to the hospital with Della. Even now, after a close shave, a cold shower and a fresh shirt and chinos, he could still feel the itch of her under his skin. The infuriating woman needled him like no other and always had. Of course, she was also mind-blowingly sexy.

'...and this is our emergency department, as you know,' said Dr Tora, Pacific Health Hospital's clinical chief of surgery, drawing Harvey away from memories of that one night three years ago when, after socialising with her family, Della had shocked him with a goodbye kiss to the cheek that had turned...explosive. As explosive as the back-and-forth bickering that had always been their main form of communication.

Forcing his head back into the game, Harvey waved hello to a few of the ED staff he recognised from his previous visits. He was proud to continue his support of this hospital. The last thing he needed was for his long-standing discord with Della to tarnish the reputation he'd built over the years.

Just then, Dr Tora's pager sounded. The older man silenced it and read the display. 'Oh dear. I'm afraid I have to go. Can I entrust Dr Wilton's security pass to you? I'm sure she'll be here soon.'

'Of course.' Harvey took the lanyard as if it were a live snake and slipped it into his pocket. Where was Della? His entire reason for meeting her at the airport was to try and mitigate any awkwardness. Since that night they'd had sex, they'd seen each other maybe six times, always in the presence of the other Wiltons. Instead, she'd fried his brain with that sexy little sundress she'd been wearing. Her blond hair was longer that the last time he'd seen her, the cut somehow softer so it fell in waves around her stunning heart-shaped face. But roaring attraction aside, they'd slipped so effortlessly into their respective roles—hers of barely concealed annoyance and his goading out those flashes of fire from her blue eyes—that clearing the air before they headed to the hospital had completely fled his mind. Images of her naked on top of him and under him, her defiant stare judging him even as she cried out in pleasure, had flashed before his eyes. They'd never once talked about that night, simply pretended that it hadn't happened. But as he'd said to her in the car, like it or not, they were stuck with each other. They'd need to find some way of putting all of that aside to work to-gether. Harvey winced, braced for a very long fortnight.

A rushed patter of feet caused him and Dr Tora to turn around. Out of breath, Della appeared. Still flus-tered. Still scowling at Harvey. Still sexy as hell. Harvey groaned silently, calling to mind how she always looked at him as if he was something unsavoury she'd found on the bottom of her shoe to manage the constant temptation.

'Sorry I'm late,' she said, addressing Dr Tora and com-pletely ignoring Harvey. 'I got a little lost.' She laced her lovely smile with apology as she stuck out her hand. 'I'm Della Wilton from Auckland's Harbour Hospital. Thank you so much for having me here at Pacific Health.'

Like Harvey, Della had obviously showered and changed since he'd dropped her at the staff bungalows an hour ago. She smelled fantastic, like an ocean breeze, her simple sleeveless dress doing nothing to hide her sensational body, not that Harvey needed a road map. He possessed an excellent memory, and he'd had nearly twenty years to study Della's abundant plus points.

'Bula, Dr Wilton,' Dr Tora said. 'I'm afraid you've just missed the tour of the surgical department, and I must excuse myself. I have an urgent referral patient to see. But I'll leave you in Dr Ward's capable hands. He knows his way around like a local after all these years.'

With a warm smile, Dr Tora departed, leaving Harvey and Della to what would no doubt be another polite and impersonal conversation, as was their norm.

'After all these years?' she asked, eyeing him suspiciously, as if he'd deliberately ruined her holiday with his presence. Her cheeks were flushed from rushing, the pale freckles on her nose a major distraction. He had intimate knowledge that they matched the ones across her shoulders and chest. Thinking about her freckles led to thinking about her naked, her gorgeous curves revealed for his greedy stare and hands. Her shockingly wild passion that, no matter how hard he tried, or how fiercely they argued, he just couldn't forget. They were like oil and water, incompatible but still flammable.

Harvey silently counted to five before opening his mouth in the hopes that he wouldn't say the wrong thing that would lead to another bickering match. The day they'd met, he'd still been grieving the death of his one and only girlfriend, Alice, sleeping around to numb the pain. Then, reeling from his instant and inconvenient attraction to his best friend's sister, he'd made some clumsy, thoughtless and cynical comment that Della and her long-distance boyfriend likely wouldn't survive them studying in different cities, in different states. Della had never forgiven him. Over the years, she took every opportunity to point out that, when it came to relationships, they wanted very different things, and her way was better.

'I come here every year,' he said, leading the way to the emergency department staff room. 'I usually run a few update seminars for our Fijian colleagues, do a few surgeries to help out.' It wasn't like he had a partner or family to holiday with, and he'd always preferred to keep busy.

'Of course you do,' she scoffed, her kissable mouth pursed with irritation. 'Why is it that you're everywhere I look, Harvey—invited to *my* family functions, working *my* job in Melbourne and now hijacking *my* holiday?'

'I could say that you followed me, Della,' he pointed out, his stare drawn to the elegant slope of her neck, a place he remembered the skin was soft and fragrant. 'It's not like I came to Fiji this year with the sole purpose of rattling your cage.'

'I wouldn't put it past you,' she muttered, walking off.

Harvey dragged in a deep breath. How would he survive two weeks in her company when they could barely make it through one conversation before she took umbrage or he goaded her? Should he remind *little miss high and mighty* how she'd used him for rebound sex three years ago, after her divorce?

Following, he caught up with her outside the occupied staff room where several nurses were taking a break. 'So, this is the ED staff room,' he said, biting his tongue for the sake of harmony. 'And this is the doctors' office.' Across the corridor, they found the office empty and stepped inside. 'Computer terminals, printers, photo-copier, etc.' Harvey slipped his hand into his pocket and pulled out her security pass. 'Use this to log in to the computer and printer.'

She took it, her expression wary.

Harvey scanned his own pass over the digital display in pointless demonstration. Della was a consultant trauma surgeon in New Zealand's leading hospital. She was per-fectly capable of figuring out how to use a photocopier. Enough procrastinating. Time to have that tricky per-sonal conversation.

'So, how have you been?' he asked, shoving his hands in his trouser pockets to appear relaxed and non-threatening. Better to get the sex talk out of the way before they started work.

'Oh, you know…' she said, moving around the room, away from him, as she pretended to scrutinise the post-ers on the notice board. 'Still the same old Della—still divorced, still working in Auckland.'

She always did that when she felt threatened—pointed out what she considered to be her worst failings, as if saying them aloud first, before anyone else could, was a defence mechanism. Not that Harvey had been about to raise either of those touchy subjects. He wasn't stupid.

'Look, Della,' he said, pushing the office door closed to give them a bit of privacy. 'I collected you from the airport because I wanted to clear the air.' He stepped into her line of vision so she couldn't ignore him. 'I know we've never talked about that night, but it was just sex.'

Just sex. The kind that had forever altered his perception and awareness of this woman. For sixteen years he'd successfully fought his attraction to her, thinking of her only as the untouchable sister of his best friend, a feat for which he surely deserved some sort of gold medal.

'There's no need to allow it to interfere with us working together for the next two weeks,' he finished, keeping his stare locked with hers. Because to look at her body was to remember that night and the way it had lit some sort of primed fuse and changed everything. Since then, there was no ignoring Della, his only defence to keep reminding himself that she was a relationship person and he was the opposite.

'As if,' she scoffed, a telltale flush creeping up her neck. 'I'm a professional, and it wasn't *that* good.'

'Liar,' he said simply, daring her with his eyes to argue the point so he could bring up how they'd set the bed ablaze, how she'd come twice and left his place looking sexily satisfied, if a little dazed. But then she'd confessed he'd been her first since her marriage had broken down six months earlier. Thinking about how she'd used *good old Harvey* to get over her ex that night, his stomach twisted. He hadn't realised how much it had bothered him until the next day when he'd awoken with the scent of her perfume on his sheets. He'd wanted to call her so badly, he'd locked his phone in the filing cabinet at work.

But Della hadn't finished insulting him.

'Well, there's no need to worry that I'll tempt you to break your *one time and done* rule,' she said, her expression withering.

She'd always made it clear what she thought of Harvey's commitment avoidance, always judged him and stuck up for the women he slept with and looked at him as if he was some kind of dirt bag. Of course, she had no idea that keeping his brief relationships superficial was how Harvey dealt with the losses in his life. Both his mother and Alice had left him in their different ways, and he never wanted there to be a third woman who made him feel powerless. He was better off alone and in control.

Harvey shook his head in disbelief, her jibe predictable but no less offensive. 'I'm not worried, and I don't have a *one time and done* rule.' He almost wished he did. That way he absolutely wouldn't be thinking about sleeping with Della again.

And was it his fault that Della was a relationship person, and with the exception of Alice, he was a bit of a loner? Was it his fault they shared a competitive streak, that they were professionally similar but personally opposites? She'd grown up surrounded by the loving but boisterous Wilton family, whereas Harvey's mother had abandoned him when he was eight years old. Was it his fault that, over the years, Harvey had deliberately stayed single whereas Della had fallen in and out of love with several unworthy men who'd one by one broken her too-big heart?

'And yet you're forty-two and have never been in a relationship that lasts longer than a bottle of milk,' she said, that curl of contempt tugging at her gorgeous mouth.

'Why do you always do that?' he asked, once more questioning the wisdom of coming to Fiji as planned once he'd discovered from Brody that Della would also be there.

'Do what?' She put one hand on her hip as if deliberately taunting him with her spectacular figure.

'Insinuate that my sex life bothers you?' He took a half step closer, his pulse accelerating as her pupils dilated, as if their bickering was a kind of verbal foreplay. 'Being sceptical about love isn't a crime, Della. And it didn't seem to matter when you needed a quick roll in the hay to celebrate the granting of your divorce order.'

She might despise his lifestyle, see him as some sort of threat because their views on commitment were so dissimilar, but she couldn't deny their rampant chemistry.

'It *doesn't* bother me,' she said, her breaths coming a little faster and her cheeks reddening. 'And don't act as if you hoped us sleeping together three years ago would be the start of something more. That's not your style.'

She was right. Just because they were trapped there together, he'd be a fool to act on this, a fool to do anything but ignore it as usual.

'So? You knew what you were getting into that night and wanted me anyway,' he pointed out. 'Perhaps because you needed a safe bet, and good old Harvey was available.' It was a low blow, but he couldn't stop himself from taunting her, not when she was acting so…holy. Not when she'd used him and never mentioned it again. Had she even given that night a second thought over the past three years?

Her mouth hung open and she blinked up at him, maybe searching for something cutting to say. But Harvey had already exposed too much. He didn't want her to know he'd been aware that he'd served a purpose that night. That her using him had stung. Maybe he could exact a little revenge now.

Stepping closer, he lowered his voice. 'Perhaps you like the idea of spending another night in my bed, Della. If that's the case, you only have to ask. For you, my bedroom door is always open.'

'Of course it is,' she muttered, triumph glittering in her wide stare. 'Same old Harvey. You never change.'

'Neither do your judgements,' he said, tempted to exaggerate stories of his past philandering for maximum effect. 'But as you've raised the subject of relationships, you obviously want me to ask. So, are *you* seeing anyone? Is husband-to-be number two waiting for you back in Auckland?'

Harvey clamped his runaway mouth shut. He didn't want to upset her any more than he already had just by being there. But a twist of envy gripped his gut. He shouldn't care if she was dating again. It was none of his business. All he needed to do was get through these two weeks in one piece.

Della raised her chin, her eyes dipping, but not before Harvey spied a flash of doubt. So that was *no* then. Hell… it would be so much easier for him if she was dating and therefore untouchable again.

'I've been busy…' she confirmed, glancing away. 'Moving countries, starting a new job, travelling home to Melbourne to visit my family every chance I get.'

Another dig about the Melbourne job… But now, fingers of unease slithered up Harvey's spine. Was she talking about the past three and a half years?

'So no dating at all since your divorce?' he pushed, the pitch of his voice changing to incredulous. Did that mean she hadn't slept with anyone else since she'd slept with *him*? Surely not. But now he was aflame with curiosity.

'My love life doesn't concern you,' she said primly, her stare bold.

Harvey saw red. 'Not even when you used me for sex, knowing that you were safe to walk away and never mention it again, despite the fact that we see each other all the time?' Now why had he said that? Why couldn't he have handed over her security pass, ignored how badly he wanted to kiss her and kept his mouth shut? Why was it these days, since that one hot night, he and Della always seemed to have some sort of unfinished business?

Her mouth agape, she blinked up at him, breathing hard.

His own heart rate thundering, his gaze dipped to the lovely curve of her lips. He knew how those lips tasted, recalled how they parted on breathy sighs. Had felt them against his skin as she'd cried out in passion. The metallic taste of fear coated his mouth. Forget the awkwardness; it wasn't their biggest problem. He wasn't going to survive these two weeks, fourteen long days, in Della's company without cracking and doing something stupid. Perhaps he should just kiss her now, suggest they sleep together again and get the sex out of their systems so they could go back to bickering over nothing.

Just then, as they faced each other, head-to-head, stares locked in defiance, there was a knock at the door. They stepped away from each other as Seema, one of the ED nurses, entered the room.

'Harvey, we've just had a walk-in casualty, and it looks bad—can you come?'

'Of course,' Harvey said, rushing to the trauma bay in the ED with Della at his heels. All the adrenaline he'd prepared for sparring with Della fuelled him now as he joined the man being wheeled on a stretcher into the re-suscitation bay.

'His work colleagues literally carried him in,' Seema said about the patient, who was conscious and groaning in pain, his breathing harsh behind an oxygen mask. 'He fell from second-floor scaffolding, a drop of over twenty feet. His name is Warren.'

Harvey glanced at Della as he reached for a stetho-scope. Their reckoning would have to wait. As if they were used to working together, she took up position op-posite Harvey, on the other side of the patient, reach-ing for a second stethoscope, as the nurses cut away the man's clothing to expose his chest. Harvey noted his vital signs. His blood pressure was on the low side, his heart rate rapid but regular.

'He has an open fracture of the left humerus,' Della said, her eyes meeting Harvey's in silent communication.

Their casualty would be heading to theatre, but first they needed to eliminate anything more life-threatening than a broken arm.

'Any loss of consciousness or seizures?' Harvey asked Seema, testing the man's pupillary reflexes with a pen torch. They needed to exclude a head injury. Fortunately someone had fitted a neck brace to immobilise the man's cervical spine.

'No,' Seema said. 'One of the work colleagues who brought him in was on the ground and got to him pretty quickly.'

'I just need to examine you, Warren.' Harvey pal-pated the trachea above the breast bone before plac-ing his stethoscope over the lung fields to listen to the breath sounds.

'He's got a pneumothorax on the left and tracheal deviation,' he told Della, knowing she would understand the urgency of the man's condition. In cases of tension pneumothorax, if they didn't drain out the escaped air from his chest and reinflate the collapsed lung, he could go into shock.

Della nodded, reaching for a sterile wide-bore cannula from the trolley at the head of the casualty. They needed to relieve the pressure on the heart by allowing the trapped air to escape before they could organise X-rays or they risked cardiac arrest.

'I think he might have a flail chest on this side,' Della said, adding to the list of problems. 'There's a lot of bruising of the chest wall and some surgical emphysema.' She peeled open the cannula as the blood pressure monitor emitted an ear-piercing alarm.

'His blood pressure is dropping. Let's decompress and then review,' he said to Della, who quickly swabbed the skin and inserted the needle into the man's chest cavity to allow the trapped air from the punctured lung to escape.

Harvey drew up some intravenous analgesia and, as the blood pressure rose, administered it via a cannula in the patient's arm. 'Warren. We think you might have some fractured ribs that have punctured the lung. We're going to organise some X-rays to be sure.'

'Let's get a chest drain kit ready, please,' Della said to Seema. 'And we need an urgent cross-match for blood transfusion.' She quickly labelled some blood vials and handed them to a porter, who would run them around to the haematology lab.

With the patient stabilised for now, Harvey and Della

moved aside to talk, their personal grievances and the constant pull of attraction set aside.

'That humerus will need to be internally fixed,' Della said with a frown of concern, shifting to make room for the radiographer, who wheeled in the mobile X-ray machine.

'We might need to surgically stabilise the fractured ribs, too,' Harvey said, his mind racing through the worst-case scenarios for the patient. Often, a flail segment, an area of ribs fractured in more than one place, was treated with mechanical ventilation and analgesia, but in some instances, surgery was required, especially if there were other complications like chest wall damage, haemorrhage or rib dislocations.

Della nodded in agreement. 'I'll call the anaesthetist and theatre. Either way, he'll need to be admitted to ICU.'

'And I'll speak to Warren's next of kin and consent him for surgery,' Harvey said, impressed with the way they'd forgotten their personal differences and their competitive natures and worked together for the first time.

'I didn't expect to operate on our first day.' She looked up at him, a flicker of surprise and respect shining in her eyes. 'Do you want the humerus or the chest?'

'Let's figure it out together when we get to theatre,' he said, confident that Della and he could set aside everything else when it came to their work.

'Sounds like a plan,' she said, her expression registering relief.

Before they found themselves trapped together in Fiji, he'd have been convinced they would squabble over the decision or over who was the better surgeon. But when it came to the safety of their patient, there was no room for ego, despite how he'd teased her earlier at the airport.

As they set about their different tasks, putting their patient first, Harvey wondered how long their enforced truce would last. Their sexual chemistry was obviously going nowhere. They would need to revisit the conversation on how best to manage it, providing they could tolerate each other long enough to talk.

As predicted, it was going to be the longest fortnight of Harvey's life.

CHAPTER THREE

LATER THAT NIGHT, after a full afternoon of surgery, Della took her frosty glass of beer from the barman and headed outside. Savu's, a beach bar a short walk from the hospital, had a handful of tables set on the sand. What better way to unwind than watching the stunning Fijian sun set. After her eventful and unexpected first day, she desperately needed time to put everything into perspective. Like how she'd almost kissed Harvey Ward earlier in the emergency department doctors' office…

What the hell had she been thinking? She'd had her 'roll in the hay', as he'd put it. The shameful memory of his hurt expression returned. He'd accused her of using him for sex that night, which she probably had on some level. But surely Harvey wouldn't have cared, would he? The man was a walking one-night stand. But maybe tomorrow, she should apologise.

Della stepped outside and instantly spied Harvey sitting alone at one of the tables near the water's edge. Her stomach swooped at the sight of him—long legs stretched out as he relaxed, his fingers casually gripping a beer bottle, his gaze trained on the ocean view. Della froze, her first instinct to forget her apology and avoid him, as usual. She could duck back inside the bar, down her beer and scurry home to her accommodation without having to analyse just how badly she still wanted the annoyingly arrogant man, despite the fact she had to work with him for the next two weeks and he still knew how to push all of her buttons.

For you, my bedroom door is always open... Right—for her and every other single woman on the planet.

As if he'd heard her scoff, he turned, and their eyes met. Della's body flushed from head to toe with that familiar jolt of attraction. Dammit, she couldn't run away now that he'd seen her, but nor did she particularly want to talk to him. If they somehow managed a conversation without bickering or hurling insults, she might feel compelled to admit that she'd found new respect for him as a doctor.

They'd spent hours in theatre with their fall casualty, internally fixing the man's fractured humerus and multiple rib fractures. To her confusion, she'd learned that Harvey was far from arrogant in the OR. When it came to surgery, he was meticulously thorough. He'd even shown humility, asking for her preferred surgical technique when it came to wiring versus plating of rib fractures.

Harvey casually raised his hand, beckoning her to join him, an easy, perfectly amicable smile tugging at that delicious mouth of his. How could he be so unaffected by her when she was all over the place? Hot with resentment that, when it came to getting over that night they'd slept together, Harvey had easily cruised into first place, leaving Della second best, she begrudgingly crossed the sand in his direction. Maybe she was simply stressed out by the idea of having him around 24-7. They'd spent more one-on-one time together today than they'd spent in the preceding nineteen years of their strained relationship. Normally, they tolerated each other for an evening maximum, and the social contact was always diluted by the presence of the other Wiltons.

As she arrived at his table, Harvey stood, pulling out the second chair. 'Great minds think alike.'

His smile, the way he swept his gaze over her, tripled her pulse rate. Why was he always so comfortable in his skin? Why did everything he did and said annoy her, so she came out fighting? Why did he have to go and show her what an all-round good guy he was, regularly donating his time and expertise here in Fiji? It was seriously messing with those preconceived assumptions she'd always clung to in order to keep Harvey in a nice, neat box.

'Yes, that was quite the first day.' Della sat and took a hasty sip of her drink, struggling anew with the surge of undeniable attraction. 'I needed to unwind.' Fat chance of that now...

'No place better than Savu's.' He smiled and raised his bottle in a toast. 'To beautiful Fijian nights.'

See, there he went again, being...nice. Della reluctantly clinked her glass to his bottle, her stomach fluttering as his stare held hers while he took a long, lazy swallow. He was so sexy, it wasn't fair. Perhaps she should sleep with him again and get it out of her system. Three years without sex really was too long—maybe when she returned to New Zealand, she should seriously consider dating again.

Jealous that she couldn't feel as unaffected by him as he appeared by her, Della scrabbled around for something to say that wasn't *I'd like to take you up on your offer and push open that bedroom door.*

'I checked on our fall patient before I left the hospital,' she said instead. 'He's stable and comfortable on ICU.'

'I checked too.' Harvey's eyes narrowed a fraction, that smug hint of amusement touching his lips, telling Della he could easily read her mind and sense her discomfort. 'But do you really want to talk shop when we could be enjoying the sunset?'

He inclined his head towards the pink-orange streaks in the sky, which deeply contrasted with the blackening sea and the patch of white sand illuminated by the lights strung overhead from the rear of the bar. Della pressed her lips together defiantly. If they couldn't talk about work, what the hell were they going to discuss? Maybe simply getting physical again was the *only* answer.

'How's Brody?' she asked, chugging another gulp of her drink, irritated by how effortlessly he could turn her on. Yes, talking about her family would smother the flames of their chemistry. Especially when it reminded her that, if not for Harvey, she would be working in Melbourne, where she belonged.

'Don't you know?' he asked, that mocking little half smile keeping her on her guard. 'He's *your* brother.'

'But you see more of him than I do,' she whined, dragging her stare away from the open neck of his shirt to where she knew his chest and torso was an anatomist's dream of sun-bronzed skin and delineated muscle. She offered him a tight smile. 'Since you stole my Melbourne job.'

She really needed to let this feud go; it was childish. And if he hadn't hijacked the lovely working holiday she'd planned, if he hadn't goaded her into talk of their sex lives, if she hadn't almost kissed him again, maybe she could have.

'Brody is good,' Harvey said with a small sigh. 'He and Amy are busy with work, but looking forward to baby Jack's naming day celebration.'

Della nodded, her heart full of longing to see her baby nephew again. She didn't need to ask if Harvey was invited to the Wilton family gathering in a month's time. He was invited to most events. Like she'd pointed out earlier, there was no escaping him.

'Look, Della, about the job...' he continued, turning serious. 'I wanted to explain. I don't know if Brody mentioned it, but my dad hasn't been well these past couple of years. I applied for that position because I really needed to stay in Melbourne. I'm all the family he has.'

Stunned by his vulnerable admission, Della shook her head in confusion. 'I didn't know. Brody never mentioned it. What's wrong with Bill?' She knew Harvey's parents were divorced and that he was close to his father. But Harvey had never opened up to her before, nor vice versa, as if they'd made an unspoken pact to keep each other at arm's length. Brody was adamant his friend had *hidden depths*, but until this very moment, she'd always doubted their existence.

'He's fine.' Harvey shrugged, clearly worried about Bill Ward but downplaying it. 'He's been diagnosed with multiple sclerosis,' he continued, his voice emotionless but his fingers picking at the corner of the beer label.

Shocked, her face heating because of how petulantly she'd acted when she hadn't known the full story, Della's throat tightened. Poor Bill. Harvey's dad was often included in family get-togethers at Christmas or on Australia Day. Della liked him a lot.

'I'm so sorry to hear that, Harvey.' Before she'd even realised she'd moved, Della found her hand resting on Harvey's warm, muscular forearm. Her comforting gesture spread tingles up her own arm. She pulled her hand away. Touching him was a no-no if she hoped to keep their sexual chemistry under control. And if Harvey could successfully ignore it, so could she.

'You must be worried about him,' she pushed, instinct telling her that control freak Harvey was probably in denial. Not that she could blame him. No one wanted to think of their parents ageing or becoming sick.

Harvey shrugged, pulling a deep drag of beer from the bottle. 'Dad's a proud man. He doesn't want pity, and he hates me fussing. But you can understand why I wanted to stay close at hand, in case he…needs me.'

'Of course…' she said, yet another of Della's rock-solid assumptions where this man was concerned disintegrating. 'Is he badly affected?'

He looked away, focused on the setting sun, as if he no longer wanted to talk about it. 'He's still managing his activities of daily living, but he struggles with the stairs. I've moved his bed to the ground floor, but ideally, I'd like him to sell up and move into an adapted bungalow.'

Della stayed silent, understanding both sides of the argument. Bill would fiercely cling to his independence, and as an only child, Harvey just wanted peace of mind that his father was safe.

'Anyway…' he said, dragging out the word to herald a change of subject. 'Back to my earlier question, before we were interrupted by our emergency. No dates in three and half years? How's that working out for you?'

Della sighed. Jerk Harvey was back. Only she could no longer hate him for beating her to her dream job, and she still needed to apologise for using him for sex. At this rate, with her justifications dissolving before her eyes, she risked becoming his...*friend.* No, the attraction would always get in the way of that. But now that she had to let go of her bitterness over losing the position to Harvey, she realised how she'd used it as a shield from thinking about that incredible night when she'd learned the stories about Harvey were true. He *was* good at everything.

'No need to sound so astounded,' she said haughtily. 'It's not fatal. I'm not ready for another relationship yet.' The last thing she wanted to discuss with Harvey was the breakdown of her marriage, the mistake she'd made in trusting Ethan, the humiliation of her divorce, when all she wanted was to be like her brother: happily married and starting a family.

'Who said anything about relationships?' Harvey asked, his stare holding hers the way it had in the ED doctors' office before they attended to the emergency, as if he could see straight through her to all her failings and weaknesses. 'I'm talking about sex.'

He took another swallow of beer and licked his lips the way Della wanted to. She swallowed, her throat bone-dry with lust. Harvey was the last man on Earth she wanted to discuss her sad lack of a sex life with.

His stare narrowed, his scrutiny making her flustered. 'So, are you saying that *your* last time was *our* last time?' he asked, incredulous.

'What if it was?' Della snapped, all the empathy she'd

felt for him a moment ago evaporating. 'You can't make a competition out of my personal life, Harvey.'

Because he'd win that argument, too. With that single exception, when she'd succumbed to Harvey Ward's charms, she'd lived like a nun since her divorce. It wasn't healthy, but Della had always needed an emotional connection to even think about being intimate with someone. That didn't make her a prude, just a woman.

'But you can make a joke out of *my* personal life?' he asked, his expression as calm as the sea before them. 'I like sex. Don't you?'

She felt his observation all over her body. Of course she liked sex. Why was that question so arousing and tempting, as if it was an offer?

'Don't goad me,' she snapped, 'just because we're different. I'm not like you.'

She looked away, hot and bothered. Why did she always allow him to get to her like this? Why couldn't she simply ignore him the way she'd tried to over the years? Because when it came to Brody's best friend, it had always been easier to dismiss and avoid him than to admit his relationship self-sufficiency, his easy-breezy attitude to dating, his cynicism about love only highlighted their differences and made Della feel somehow inadequate, reigniting those fears that she was being left behind in her family. She'd always wanted a loving, committed relationship and a family of her own, whereas Harvey didn't even believe in love.

But there was no chance of ignoring him now that they had to spend the best part of the next two weeks working together. No wonder she was feeling volatile.

'In what way are we different?' he asked, appearing

genuinely curious. 'I think we have a surprising amount in common, considering we're always arguing.'

Della dragged in a deep breath. She wanted to point out that *he* was responsible for their bickering, but she held back. They were finally going to have a meaningful conversation, after all the years of avoiding it with polite smiles and impersonal comments and, on Della's part, cowardice and self-preservation.

'Oh, come on, Harvey,' she said warily, 'we're total opposites, especially when it comes to relationships. And don't pretend that we could ever get along. You've never even liked me.'

Harvey took another lazy swallow of beer, his eyes on hers. 'I like you just fine, Della.'

The husky drawl of his voice turned her limbs molten with desire. Was that true? Did he like her? Admitting that he might be telling the truth, that Harvey did have another, deeper side, sat like a rock in her stomach, reminding her how she *had* used him for sex that night and he'd probably not only known it but also felt hurt.

'If you like me so much,' she said, on the attack, jittery with nerves from his admission, 'why take the moral high ground when it comes to our differences? To relationships? It's as if you see the kind of commitment most people want, the kind *I* want, as some sort of threat. As if you're too smart to fall in love like the rest of us, or you think love is a joke.'

'I don't think that at all,' he said, looking mildly uncomfortable for the first time. 'We've just always wanted different things. But you've done your fair share of judging, Della, right from the moment we met.'

'Well, you insulted me,' she said, aware she was overreacting and dragging up ancient history. 'We'd just been introduced, and you felt comfortable enough to point out my relationship at the time was doomed. In fact, you've objected to every one of my past boyfriends for some reason or another,' she continued. 'You didn't even like Ethan, as if *you,* the great relationship expert, Harvey Ward, were somehow privy to inside knowledge that our marriage wouldn't last.' She hated that he'd been right, *again*. That unlike Della, he'd shown good judgement when it came to her ex. No wonder she wasn't ready to trust her intuition and risk another relationship just yet. Perhaps she should take a leaf out of Harvey's book and enjoy a casual sexual fling.

'And you've always objected to *me,*' he said, eyes glittering. 'As if I wasn't a good enough friend for Brody or good enough to be associated with your family, just because I prefer to be single.'

Della sat back in outrage. 'See, this always happens. We're fooling ourselves if we expect to make it through two weeks of working together. We're too different, too competitive to ever get along.' She glugged a mouthful of beer, looking away from him in disgust. The Wiltons were an ambitious bunch, and Harvey fit right in. Della had struggled growing up in golden boy Brody's exalted footsteps, and then, just when she'd started to make her own mark by getting into medical school, he'd brought home driven, talented Harvey.

'We can do it if we have to,' he said calmly, where Della was braced for another battle. 'We didn't argue that night in bed. Or have you forgotten?'

Despite her temper, Della's body incinerated. She scowled at him. 'How could I forget when over the years

I've heard so many wild stories of your sex life from Brody?' She leaned forward, needing to win this argument. 'The threesomes. The heartbroken women past their expiration dates. Your rotating bedroom door and your untouchable heart.'

Harvey's lip curled, his stare narrowing as he watched her with curiosity. 'It was *one* threesome, and that was years ago.' His dark gaze rested on her lips. 'But you sound jealous, Della. We can rectify that.' He spread his arms wide and relaxed back in the chair in a *come and get me* gesture.

Every cell in her body perked up, his offer beyond tempting. How would she fight this physical compulsion for two whole weeks? Not even them bickering seemed to douse the flames. 'Oh please...' Della scoffed, her body temperature high with irritation and fierce desire. 'I am *so* done with men.'

Of course, he was right; they were good together. Great, in fact. A big part of her wanted another go at Harvey if for no other reason than to wipe that smug look off his face.

'Hey,' Harvey said, holding up a hand to ward off her unfair comparison, 'don't go bringing your ex into this again.' He took another swig of beer, cool, calm and collected.

Della dragged in a ragged breath. She was being overemotional. She didn't care one jot if Harvey slept with every other woman on the planet *but* her. Time to change the subject.

'Why didn't you like Ethan,' she asked, a lump in her throat, 'just out of interest?' She shouldn't care; her marriage and divorce were *her* business. But the part of her that had always compared herself to golden boy Brody and then later to carefree Harvey was scared to completely trust her own judgement. Had she missed some sign that others had seen? Ethan had wooed her with a whirlwind romance, proposed after a couple of years and then slowly changed once they were married. And Della hadn't seen the divorce coming.

'Let's not go there.' Harvey instantly sobered, glancing away. 'It's in the past, and it's nothing to do with me.' He clenched his jaw as if he had no intention of answering her question.

'Come on, I want to know,' Della pushed, her curiosity so wild, her heart rate went through the roof. It must be bad if he was refusing to say. Hot shame washed through her. It was bad enough that she'd failed at something Brody had nailed—a successful marriage and a family. Even worse that Harvey, of all people, had witnessed Della's defeat and now seemed to have some kind of insider knowledge.

'Leave it, Della.' Harvey frowned as he made eye contact, warning in his stare. 'You won't like what I have to say. We'll end up arguing again.'

'Tell me anyway,' she demanded, embarrassment a head-to-toe itchy rash. 'I insist.' Had there been some glaringly obvious flaw in her and Ethan's relationship? Had outsiders deduced what Della herself hadn't seen coming? Had Harvey correctly predicted that her marriage had been doomed?

With a sigh, Harvey reluctantly surrendered. 'I've known you since you were eighteen, Della. You wear your big heart on your sleeve. Fall in love and dive in, as if... I don't know. As if you somehow have something to prove. As if you're in competition with every other couple out there.'

Della gasped, mortified. 'I've also grown up since you first met me, Harvey.' Although she couldn't help but compare herself to her brother. She shrank inside, feeling sick. How dare untouchable Harvey, her nemesis, know her so well. How dare he see her need to be loved and to be accepted as she was so effortlessly when he didn't know the first thing about the emotion. Could he also see her deepest fear, that by pushing for a family, she'd pushed Ethan away?

'Trust me,' she continued with a scoff, bluffing for all she was worth, 'I have no interest in exposing my heart or diving into another relationship until I'm certain the lucky guy wants exactly what *I* want.'

She'd learned her mistake with Ethan. At the end, he'd accused her of being *baby obsessed*, even though when they'd met, he'd said he too wanted a family. But next time she was ready for a relationship, it would be with someone who, like her, wanted it all: commitment, marriage, a family. Yet how could she ever be certain they were being truthful when Ethan had managed to dupe her?

'Good...' Harvey shrugged, his expression full of regret as if he hated what he was about to say. 'Because sometimes...little things he said... I just got the impression that Ethan was... I don't know...holding something back.'

Della froze, wishing she hadn't asked but some sick twisted part of her willing him to continue.

'When you got engaged,' he said, his stare searching

hers, 'I genuinely hoped for your sake that I was wrong. That it would work out. That you'd be happy.'

Her eyes stung. She absolutely must not cry in front of Harvey. *Never ever.* Because he was right. When they'd met and fallen in love, Ethan had claimed he'd wanted the same things. But once they'd married, once they'd fallen into a routine of work and sharing a home, he'd started putting off their conversations about starting a family, made her feel as if the dream was suddenly one-sided. He'd used her desire to have it all to make her feel that *his* job was more important. Shamefully, she'd followed him to Sydney so he could pursue *his* career, reasoning that someone had to compromise. But even after his big promotion, he'd continued to put off talk of kids. Della had given the marriage her all, and delayed becoming a mother while Ethan established himself in an ortho-paedic consultant role, but it hadn't been enough. He'd come home one day and said he wasn't ready to be a fa-ther and left. And Della had been blindsided. But *Harvey*, a man who knew nothing about relationships, had somehow predicted it.

Returning to the present, Della blinked, shivered, chilled to the bone. Harvey's concerned face came back into focus, something like pity in his stare. Her stomach turned with sickening humiliation.

'Well, bravo, Harvey—you were right, again,' she said, shame and failure a fire in her blood. 'You, who don't even believe in love, saw my marriage the way it truly was. But then, you'd know all about holding back, wouldn't you? You've never had a relationship. Do you even possess a heart, Harvey? Or are all those messy human emotions for the rest of us poor misguided fools?'

How could she have been so stupid as to consider sleeping with him again? They were polar opposites, too competitive and threatened by each other to ever see eye to eye. They couldn't even have one simple conversation.

'I don't think that,' he said, reaching for her arm.

But the damage was done. Della snatched it out of his reach. Rising to her feet, she shoved the seat back so hard, it toppled to the sand. 'I'll see you tomorrow,' she said, for once her voice staying impressively calm. 'Can I suggest that, for the sake of harmony, to make the next two weeks even remotely bearable, that we restrict our conversations to work, after all.' Without waiting for an answer, she stomped off.

CHAPTER FOUR

DELLA ENTERED HER staff bungalow on the hospital grounds and slammed the door. The reverberations jolted through Harvey from his position across the street. He'd followed her, of course. He'd never have been able to sleep if he hadn't made certain she'd arrived home safely.

He dragged in a shuddering breath, guilt making him cringe. He should never have allowed himself to be lured into a personal conversation. They couldn't be trusted not to bicker, insult and upset each other. Then she'd forced him to talk about her ex, demanding he be honest, before throwing his reluctant observations back in his face.

Why could they never have a nice, normal chat? Maybe because the attraction was always there, bubbling away beneath the surface. Harvey *hadn't* liked any of her boyfriends. She was right. None of them were good enough for her, not even Ethan. She was funny and smart and would do anything for anyone, and after today, Harvey had gained a massive amount of respect for her as a surgeon.

Harvey crossed the road, regret a weight on his shoulders. What the hell did he know about committed relationships anyway? He'd been alone by choice for twenty years, after Alice had died in a car accident. He'd assumed he'd get over her death in time and want another relationship, but as the years had passed, he'd become increasingly convinced that he should have known better than to pin his happiness on another person. After all, if his own mother hadn't loved him enough to stick around, what hope did he have of finding someone with whom he could share his life?

Harvey tapped on the door to Della's bungalow, his gut twisting. The last thing he wanted to do was hurt Della. Why would she care what *he* had to say? But maybe she saw her divorce as some sort of failing, even though it was her ex who chose to leave the marriage.

The door flew open, as if she'd been standing and fuming on the other side.

'You left your sunnies at the bar,' he said, wearing an apologetic expression as he held out the sunglasses.

'Thanks.' She took them, dropping them onto the table just inside the door. When she looked at him again, her stare brimmed with hurt that he'd inadvertently put there because, ever since that night three years ago, he couldn't seem to manage this attraction.

'I'm sorry, Della,' he said, contrite. 'I didn't mean to hurt you. My comments were…thoughtless. I don't think you're a fool for falling in love. The opposite, in fact.' He stared into her blue eyes, forcing himself to open up in order to repair the damage. 'It's not that I don't believe in love. It's more that making yourself vulnerable with another person is a brave gamble. But then, I'm hardly an expert. As you pointed out, what do *I* know about relationships?'

She eyed him hesitantly, still wearing a frown.

'You shouldn't listen to me,' he went on. 'I just

wouldn't want you to be hurt again, that's all. If I'm honest, I didn't like your boyfriends because none of them were good enough for you.'

He shut his mouth, suddenly exhausted. He'd already given away how protective he felt of her, when he had no right. Her love life was none of his business, and *he* wasn't the man of anyone's dreams. At least she was brave enough to put herself out there, whereas he simply avoided the risk of letting someone close, of giving them the power to cause pain. When it came to matters of the heart, *she* was the experienced one.

Della sighed, her body relaxing. 'I *did* push for your honest opinion,' she said, shaking her head with regret. 'And I threw my fair share of insults your way. Maybe I just hate that you're always right. That, like Brody, you're better than me at *everything*.' Her lips twitched with amusement, telling him he was forgiven.

Harvey's pulse pounded with relief, but his stare raked hers. Did she compare herself unfavourably to Brody? Harvey was an only child, so he had no reference when it came to sibling rivalry.

'Not everything,' he said, a cautious smile forming. 'Definitely not relationships.' Harvey's parents had split when he was kid, so as far as he was concerned, relationship breakdowns were inevitable. Maybe it was time to tell Della about Alice, about his mother, about why the cynical twenty-three-year-old she'd met had been so down on commitment and still was, if pushed.

'Only because you've never had one,' she said, rolling her eyes. 'If you had, I'm sure that, like Brody, you'd have made it work. You'd probably be living *my* life by now—successful career, happily married, a houseful of adorable children.'

Harvey hid a wince, wishing he could say something to help reassure Della that she still had time to achieve her dreams, but he'd already overstepped the mark once tonight. He hated that she wanted what Brody had, but had been let down by her ex. Maybe once, a long time ago, Harvey might have harboured that same dream, back when he'd thought he was in control of his life and his heart. But growing up abandoned by his mother, the only woman who should have loved him unconditionally, had taught him that feelings, entrusting your happiness to another person, was a big risk. And he'd re-learned that same lesson the hard way when Alice had died.

'Well, if it's any consolation,' he said, steering the conversation back to the relative safety of work, 'having seen you in action in the OR today, I'd say you can hold your own as a surgeon with both me and Brody.' Respect for her bloomed anew. She was a good doctor and a talented surgeon, damn sexy qualities. But then, everything about Della was sexy and always had been. Probably why he goaded her. Nothing worse than forbidden fruit to increase ardour. And apart from that one lapse, when he'd kissed her back, one thing leading to another, Harvey was smart enough to stay well away. They wanted different things in life. Della wanted that marriage, husband, a houseful of kids dream, and Harvey liked being in control of his life and his emotions. So why was he struggling to walk away now?

'Careful, Harvey.' She smiled, eyed in him in that way that heated his blood, but also told him she could laugh at herself and at him. 'That sounds suspiciously like another compliment.'

He dragged in a shaky breath. 'Good. It is. Will you be okay?' He hesitated on the doorstep, needing to know that their stupid fight hadn't caused lasting damage to Della's self-esteem. He should leave. Let her get some sleep before their seminars in the morning. But he cared about her and genuinely wanted to see her happy.

'Of course.' She blinked, watched him with curiosity as if seeing him for the first time. 'I'm a strong, independent and resilient woman. It will take more than one little divorce to keep me down.'

'I know you are,' he said, seeing through her bravado. Those old protective urges resurfaced. The Harvey that had first met this woman had known all about the pain of heartbreak. It had been hard to stand on the sidelines and watch big-hearted Della go through break-up after break-up and finally her divorce. Not that looking out for her, back then or now, was his place.

'Okay... I'll...um...let you get some rest.' He took a half step back, his feet dragging. Being trapped with her in Fiji had forced him to admit how badly he still wanted her, how the grip he thought he had on his attraction was weakened because he couldn't avoid temptation and walk away the way he had three years ago, the way he did every time he'd seen her since. Nor could he shake the knowledge that she hadn't had sex with another man since him, that she still wasn't ready for a relationship. And if he needed one more sign that this trip had been sent to test him and his belief that Della was out of his system, she was looking at him in *that* way again.

'Thanks...' she said, touching his arm. 'For the sunglasses *and* the compliment. It means a lot coming from you.'

Her touch burned his skin, her words an acknowledgement that they might be different, but when it came to work, they respected each other.

'You're welcome.' His voice was scratchy. His feet didn't seem to want to move.

'You know,' she said, blinking up at him, 'I'm sorry, too.' Her breathing came faster. 'I *did* use you for sex that night. You were right about that, as well.' She blushed and Harvey shrugged it off, his pulse roaring because she was still touching his arm.

'That's okay. Truth is, I was happy to be used.' What kind of idiot would turn down sex with someone as gorgeous as Della, even if he had been her rebound? He'd never forgotten that night, probably because Della Wilton, like the rest of her loving, boisterous family, was a massive part of his life. But they really shouldn't discuss sex any more tonight or he'd never make it off this doorstep.

'I wanted to feel attractive again after, you know, being rejected,' she said, looking down and then meeting his stare. 'But it's not okay that I hurt you in the process.'

Harvey understood rejection, but were they declaring a truce? 'You're beautiful, Della. And I'm a grown man. I wanted you too much to care about your motivations.' Adrenaline rushed through his system. It felt good to admit that after all these years of pretending he didn't find her incredibly attractive. But this was dangerous territory.

Her eyes widened. Time slowed as they stared. What was it about this place that completely altered the nature of their relationship? It was as if for the first time ever they were being honest. Finally, Harvey tilted his head in resignation and stepped back. If he didn't leave now, he was going to do something stupid. And this time, there'd be no walking away, no pretending it hadn't happened, at least not until they left Fiji.

'Wait,' she said, reaching for the hem of his shirt and tugging. 'Don't go.'

He crossed the threshold. She closed the door, pulled him closer.

'Della…is this a good idea?' His hands found her waist, neither drawing her close nor holding her distant. Their bodies were inches apart. The heat of her, the subtle scent of her perfume, called to that part of him he'd always needed to lock down in her presence.

'It's just sex, Harvey,' she argued with a shrug, tossing back his earlier words. 'Best to get it out of the way so we can move on and work together, don't you think?'

Think…? All of his blood had left his brain. Thinking was impossible. But his instincts were still firing. 'I want you, but I don't want to hurt you again or give you the wrong idea about us. You know me.' They were too different for more than sex. Under all her bluff and bluster, Della was a funny, caring and wildly passionate woman any guy looking to settle down would be lucky to have. But Harvey wasn't that guy, and they both knew it.

'Come on, Harvey.' She blinked up at him, her stare dark with desire and unspoken challenge. 'I'm an intelligent woman. I'd never be stupid enough to expect anything but sex from a man like *you*.'

Reassurance dressed as an insult, but she was right. She knew him the way he knew her. He wasn't relationship material, and Della wanted it all. Of course, she didn't know everything about his past—some ugliness was too uncomfortable to share—but she knew enough to have realistic expectations.

'Are you worried that I'm using you for sex again?' she asked, a playful glint in her blue eyes. 'Because if it helps, I totally am.'

Harvey fought his instincts. He should have felt relieved that they were on the same page. That just like last time, Della wasn't looking for anything serious. But somewhere deep down, her words—*a man like you... using you for sex again*—also stung. Despite what she believed, Harvey *did* possess a heart. He'd just trained it to have very low expectations.

'I'm not worried,' he lied, clinging to reason as she inched closer, her breasts grazing his chest. He gripped her face, tilted that lovely mouth up to within a whisper of his. 'I just want you to be sure. Eyes wide open like last time.'

'I want you.' Della held his stare as she surged up on tiptoe and sought his mouth with hers. She gripped his neck and pulled him down, closing the distance. Della knew what she wanted, and she was right—this was the best way to break the tension so they could get through two weeks of forced proximity.

Too late to overthink it, Harvey crushed her close. The first touch of their kiss flooded his strung-out body with energising endorphins. Their lips parted. Tongues met, surged, tasted. A sense of déjà vu struck, as if he recalled every detail of the last time they kissed. As if they aligned perfectly.

'Harvey...' Della moaned as he slid his lips down the side of her neck.

His name on her lips shifted something primal and urgent inside him, so he pressed her body closer. Selfishly, on some level, Harvey needed to know that Della wanted him for no other reason than this fierce, immoveable attraction. This time, there was no ghost of another man to chase off. This was about *them*.

'Why is it that we get on so much better without words,' she panted, sliding her hands inside his T-shirt, her palms branding his skin.

'I have no idea.' Harvey backed her up, pressing her against the wall to increase the contact between their bodies. Maybe it was because words were open to misinterpretation, whereas physically, they just clicked. Harvey ground his hips against hers, urgency to be inside her pounding through his veins. Della angled her head, exposing her neck to his kisses. Then she shoved up his shirt, yanking it over his head and tossing it before removing her own.

He looked down to where her breasts were encased in sexy black lace. 'I swear you get sexier each time I see you.' And he was only human. Della was too sexy to ignore when she was on the other side of the room shooting him disapproving looks. Like this, seductive, needy in his arms, saying all the right things, he'd had no hope of resisting.

Kissing her again, he hoisted her from the floor so she wrapped her legs around his waist, her fingers demanding in his hair. She moaned as he cupped one breast through her bra, kissing his jaw, his neck, the notch between his collarbones while her hips undulated against his. Harvey's eyes rolled closed, the friction between their writhing bodies almost unbearable.

'Hold tight,' he said, slinging his arms under her butt and striding to the bedroom. He placed her on her feet, and she unclasped and removed her bra.

'Hurry,' she said, tugging at the waistband of his shorts. 'It's been three years.'

'Whose fault is that?' Harvey smiled as he popped the button on her sexy denim cut-off shorts, then scooped her back into his arms. Their naked chests pressed together, and he walked them back towards the bed. 'Besides, that's all the more reason not to rush.'

Ducking his head, he captured first one of her nipples in his mouth and then the other.

'See,' she gasped, her head falling back, 'you always need to be right, even now.'

'And you always need to have the last word.' He grinned, laying her down on the bed. He unzipped her shorts and slid them and her underwear down her shapely legs.

For a second he simply stared, swaying on his feet. She was glowing, beautiful, her stare heavy with desire. A knot formed under his ribs. This might be just sex, but Della was precious, almost family, as much a part of the furniture in his life as the rest of the Wiltons. He couldn't afford to mess this up just because he wanted her and the feeling was mutual.

'Don't overthink it, Harvey,' she said, holding out her hand for his. 'Just come here.'

Before he got too carried away by temptation, Harvey removed his wallet from his pocket, took out a condom and placed it on the bed. Then he kicked off his shoes and took her hand, lying down at her side.

'Kiss me,' she demanded, wrapping her arms around

his shoulders and hooking one leg over his hip so his doubts were silenced.

He cupped her backside and pushed his tongue against hers, laughing when she rolled him onto his back and sat astride him.

'So it's like that, is it?' he asked, toying with her nipples as she leaned over him to kiss him once more. He didn't mind her being on top or making demands or using him for sex. He'd grown accustomed over the years to the power play in his every interaction with Della, and he liked her playful side. She groaned as his hands skimmed her waist, her hips, guiding them to rock against his hard length.

'Stop teasing me,' she ordered, kissing him with renewed desperation.

When he rolled them again, tore his mouth from hers and trailed kisses down her neck, chest and stomach, she sighed in surrender. Going lower, he spread her thighs and covered her with his mouth. She cried out, her fingers spearing his hair. He wanted to take his time, to savour her, to unleash more of that wildly passionate Della that had blown him away three years ago. Her moans intensified. He pushed his fingers inside her and groaned as she tensed, gasped, climaxed, crying out his name once more. Triumph expanded his chest. If she'd waited three years, he wanted tonight to be memorable. She was right; this was their best form of communication. They didn't need feelings or hurtful words or one-upmanship. Just touch and honest desire.

'You are so sexy,' he said, shoving off his shorts and briefs. He rolled on the condom and kissed his way back up her satiated body.

'Don't be smug,' she whispered, smiling and breathless, drawing his mouth back to hers as she wrapped her hand around his erection.

'I'm afraid you can't stop me.' He grinned, gripped her thigh and drew it over his hip so he sank between her legs. 'Three years *is* a long time. Did you think about us?' He had.

'I might have done, on occasion,' she admitted begrudgingly, her pupils dilating as she snagged her lip with her teeth. 'But you don't need your ego stroking.'

Too late. With his heart thudding triumphantly because he hadn't been alone in reliving that night, Harvey laughed and swooped in for another kiss. Even after her orgasm, when admitting that they were hot together—that, like him, she'd struggled to forget—Della needed to come out on top. But with them naked and pleasuring each other rather than fighting, there was no point hiding how good they were together physically.

'Go slow,' she whispered, spreading her legs, inviting him into her body with a teasing tilt of her hips.

He pushed inside her, their stares locked. 'I thought about us, too,' he admitted, fighting his instincts to move.

Her eyes widened, a small gasp leaving her throat.

'Every time I saw you, I wanted you again, even while we fought and bickered and tried to pretend it hadn't happened.' He moved inside her body, his heart banging against hers.

'I wanted you, too,' she gasped as he thrust faster. Della tunnelled her fingers into his hair and drew his lips to hers, pushed her tongue into his mouth so he groaned. They'd never stood a chance of ignoring this attraction, this connection. They were too good together. Their sparks were exceptional. Fighting it was almost a crime against sex.

As he found the perfect rhythm, Harvey fought his own need. He wanted her with him, a tied race. He wanted her as consumed as him, so that they might move on, but they'd never forget.

'Harvey,' Della gasped, and he kissed her, cupped her beautiful breasts, thumbed her nipples erect and watched as desire darkened her blue eyes to navy.

'Come with me,' he said, picking up the pace so Della cried out and crossed her ankles in the small of his back, her fingernails digging into his arms. Harvey bent one knee for purchase, driving harder and faster. As fire raced down his spine, Harvey sent her tumbling over the edge once more, finally following her with a harsh groan, his body racked with spasms. He buried his face in the crook of her neck, sucked in the scent of her skin and wrung every drop of pleasure from their bodies.

Finally he released Della to collapse, satiated, at her side. They stared at the ceiling, both panting.

'Why did I wait so long?' Della asked, a satisfied smile stretching her lips.

'Beats me…' Harvey grinned. He'd been absolutely right about their unfinished business. But as the oxygen returned to his brain, awareness returned. Reason. Sense. Yes, their chemistry was still explosive, but it was also still something to be very wary of. Because neither of them had changed in the past three years. They still wanted different things when it came to relationships.

As he scooped a breathless Della into his arms, Harvey gritted his teeth, prepared for a fierce internal battle of desire for her, for *this*, versus self-preservation. Two weeks didn't feel like a long time, but if they kept being intimate, it was long enough to form a habit. When it came to relationships, he'd spent years fighting that kind of trap, keeping people out.

Surely he could survive thirteen more days until he could put some distance between himself and the temptation of Della?

CHAPTER FIVE

THE NEXT MORNING in the seminar room, Della tried to focus on Harvey's talk on sports-related trauma, but her mind kept wandering. Had last night really happened? How had they gone from arguing in Savu's to sleeping together again? Oh, she'd instigated it by asking him to stay. The minute he'd stood on the doorstep and apologised, the minute he'd opened up, let her in, hinting at his beliefs on love, the minute he'd alluded to the fact that, despite appearances, he'd always had a thing for her, all the anger and humiliation inside her had drained away.

How could she stay angry with Harvey, when she'd always had a thing for him too? When she'd seen another side to him? And how could the sex between them have been better than the last time? They'd had sex three times—the second time in the shower and again in bed before finally collapsing into a state of replete exhaustion. She'd awoken at dawn to the unfamiliar heat and sounds of a tropical island and nudged Harvey awake. He'd untangled his limbs from hers, kissed her, dressed and rushed back to his own bungalow, giving Della a brief reprieve to come to terms with the fact that Harvey seemed to be hotter than ever before.

How was that even possible, let alone fair? And what

did it mean for her attempts to resist him? Dragging her gaze from the man in question, Della glanced around the room. A small audience, predominantly doctors and physiotherapists from the hospital with a handful of local GPs, listened to Harvey talk. Della zoned back into what he was saying, their eyes briefly meeting, before he looked back down at his notes.

Shivers of both delight and dread danced down her spine. What was he thinking? Did he want this physical fling to continue for the duration of their time in Fiji, or was he done? He was giving little away, although he could hardly look at her the way he had last night in front of an audience. Della herself was horribly confused. On the one hand, having incredible sex with Harvey was better than two weeks of arguing. They were trapped there, after all. But was it wise? She'd never known Harvey to see a woman more than a few times. Would he even be up for a holiday fling? Or should they agree to put the sex behind them again and simply focus on working together? Her stomach sank at the thought. But just because she still wanted him, just because she'd witnessed a deeper side to Harvey she hadn't known existed, she'd do well to remember that when it came to relationships, they were total opposites. She sighed; she was talking herself around in circles.

The audience broke into a round of applause, and Della joined in. Harvey's talk had obviously concluded, although she'd missed most of it with her lusty daydreams.

'Thank you, Dr Ward,' Dr Tora said. 'A very informative update. We'll take a fifteen-minute break. Refreshments are available out on the veranda.'

While Harvey was approached by an audience member with a question, Della stepped outside and helped herself to a glass of iced water. There was no point trying to eat. Her stomach was too full of butterflies, her head too full of the dilemma. In theory, a little holiday sex hurt no one, especially when she and Harvey understood each other so well. At this moment, Della wasn't ready for more than sex, and even when that changed, she'd never consider Harvey. He didn't do relationships. So where was the harm in a brief sexual fling? But could she spend all this time with him, explore a sexual relationship that was obviously heading nowhere, and keep emotional boundaries in place?

'Thanks for the wake-up call,' a deep voice said over her shoulder, jolting her out of her thoughts.

Della hid a delicious shudder of anticipation, turning to offer Harvey a tight, professional smile as if they were no more than colleagues. 'You're welcome. The sunrise woke me.' Finding Harvey's big, manly body sprawled in her bed, taking up more than his fair share of space, she'd watched him sleep for a few indulgent seconds, carefully sniffing the scent of his shampoo and memorising the small scar on his shoulder. Even asleep, he was outrageously handsome.

'So…how are you feeling today?' he asked in a low voice, taking a sip of what smelled like strong black coffee, his favourite. 'Any regrets? I know I'm not your favourite person.' His voice was light as he watched her intently over the rim of his cup, his playful reminder well-timed. They'd been adversaries for so long. Could they truly be lovers, even temporarily?

'Hmm…' Della kept her expression serious and pretended to think about it. 'I guess I can live with what happened, given *I* was the one to instigate it.' She didn't want him thinking last night was his idea. 'How about you?' she asked, with a twitch of a smile. 'Have you booked the first flight out of here and deleted me from your contacts yet?'

Just because he'd admitted he'd thought all of her boyfriends including her ex-husband unworthy didn't mean their very different views on commitment and love had changed. What had he called it? A *brave gamble*? But why?

Harvey shrugged, his stare flirtatious. 'Not quite yet.'

Della fought a smile and looked down. There was a perfectly professional distance between his body and hers. To the outsider, they might be having a medicine-related conversation. Instead, her body was aflame. How could zero physical contact generate so many sparks?

'When you think about it,' she said, emboldened but her heart galloping with nerves, 'holiday flings are pretty harmless.' A safe, casual sex fling might do her a world of good. She searched his stare for any sign that he was done, although this was Harvey—short-lived flings were his forte. But if he was waiting for her to beg, he'd be waiting a long time.

'Hmm… They do have considerable benefits.' Harvey nodded, his expression thoughtful. 'A nice, neat end date when you fly home to the real world.'

Holding her nerve, she waited. She refused to crack until he cracked first. But surely they were on the same page? Surely them sleeping together benefited them working together harmoniously?

Flushed from her shameful justifications, Della held her breath as Harvey inched closer and dipped his head.

'As long as both parties use the other for the same thing, of course.'

Heartened, she caught a flicker of excitement in his eyes. Mentally, she raised a victory fist. She was willing to be used for sex, as long as she could use him in return.

'Of course. And this Fiji. Different rules apply,' she added, looking for his agreement. 'Once we leave this island, usual business resumes.'

'I agree,' he said, a small frown tugging at his mouth. 'Because we *will* see each other again.'

Della nodded, the warning clear. It was the same debate she'd been ruminating on all morning. Yes, their affair would end, but they couldn't ghost each other. Harvey would still be Brody's best friend, and Della would still see him at Wilton family functions.

'But by then,' she went on, reassuring herself as much as Harvey, 'we will have each moved on. Melbourne has a very active singles scene, I believe.' Harvey would find ample casual distractions once he returned to Australia. As they said, a leopard never changed its spots.

Harvey's stare intensified with that flicker of challenge she was used to. 'And maybe you'll find everything you want in Auckland—that devoted husband, a houseful of adorable children. You already have the successful career part.'

See, they knew each other so well. Uninvited, his words from the night before rushed Della's mind… *It's not that I don't believe in love...* Last night, she'd been too upset with him to give the statement much thought. But now it niggled at her. Was this another of Harvey's hidden depths? Was there some reason he'd sworn off relationships beyond his general cynicism following his parents' divorce?

'So, where does that leave us, I wonder?' she asked, dismissing the idea, because his motivations for staying single changed nothing. Harvey would likely never cancel his membership to the singles club, and Della still wanted it all with the right man. She wasn't stupid. There was no way she and Harvey, of all men, could be anything serious. She'd already made one big mistake with Ethan. Next time she risked her heart, she'd make sure the man was all in.

'I guess the door is still open to possibility,' he said cryptically, his stare sparking with heat, the expression doing silly things to Della's pulse. How could she still want him after last night? She'd lost count of how many orgasms she'd had, but it would be so easy to become addicted to sex that good.

'Speaking of possibility,' he said, stepping back so they were once more that respectable distance apart, 'I wondered if you'd like to explore one of the smaller islands with me later, as we have the afternoon off? We could rent a kayak and some snorkel gear. There's no point wasting the fantastic downtime opportunities.'

'That sounds good,' she said, visualising other opportunities—them alone and naked. 'As long as it's not Mallau Island,' she added with a mock grimace. 'I spent my ill-fated honeymoon there.' She offered him a wry smile, shoving all thoughts of Ethan from her mind. She'd moved on, her biggest regret that she hadn't seen through him sooner and saved herself both time and heartache.

But Harvey sobered, a small frown lodging between his brows. 'I wouldn't want to bring up any painful reminders for you. Why don't *you* choose our destination. A clean slate.'

'I will,' Della said breezily, hoping to reassure him, while enjoying that he was…protective. 'Don't look so worried. Mallau isn't the only stunning island in the archipelago.' There were over three hundred.

'In that case,' Harvey said, leaning in a little closer and dropping his voice, 'I'll do my best to keep your mind very much in the present and help you make some new memories.' The innocently phrased promise dripped with suggestion, filling Della with the thrilling fizz of anticipation.

'No, *I'll* help *you* make some,' she breathed, already looking forward to exploring Fiji with Harvey. Despite a worrying start, her working holiday had taken a very unexpected but pleasurable turn. Maybe two weeks trapped with Harvey in paradise wouldn't be so bad after all.

Just then, Dr Tora appeared from the seminar room, his face tense with concern. 'Excuse me, everyone,' he called. 'There's been a vehicle collision off the King's Road north of here. A minibus full of backpackers left the road and ploughed downhill into the dense bush. There are multiple casualties expected in the emergency department shortly. Can everyone who's available please head there to help where they can?'

As he spoke, multiple pagers sounded around them, urgent calls to their Fijian colleagues coming thick and fast.

Della and Harvey glanced at each other and abandoned their drinks. Their afternoon off, their downtime together—exploring, snorkelling, falling into bed—would have to wait. Duty called. They took off running, making it to the ED a few minutes later, in time to intercept the first wave of casualties.

'We have a twenty-three-year-old male with a penetrating abdominal wound,' the paramedic handing over a patient said as he wheeled the stretcher into a vacant resuscitation bay.

'He was flung from the window and impaled on a broken tree branch,' the paramedic continued. 'He has IV access, and I've given him morphine and IV fluids. Blood pressure is on the low side, but he's been conscious throughout.'

The casualty groaned in pain. Della sprang into action, listening to the young man's chest and abdominal sounds as nursing staff connected him to heart monitors and oxygen and began cutting away his clothing. A junior ED doctor drew blood from the man's arm to cross-match for a blood transfusion.

Harvey removed the dressing and exposed the wound in the patient's abdomen. A five-centimetre-diameter tree branch protruded from the wound just under his ribs on the right.

Della met Harvey's stare, seeing her concerns mirrored there. The risk of internal haemorrhage with injuries of this nature was high. This patient would need an urgent laparotomy to assess the internal damage and remove the branch. But if he was bleeding internally, first he must be stabilised.

'Let's get four units of blood cross-matched,' Harvey called to the junior ED doctor. 'Any sign of pneumothorax?' he asked Della, reaching for his own stethoscope.

'No,' she said, drawing up some more analgesia, 'but it will be a miracle if this has avoided his liver.'

Harvey nodded, his expression grim. They needed to operate on the man as soon as possible.

'I need an infusion of intravenous antibiotics, please,' Della said to Seema, the ED nurse, keeping one eye on the blood pressure monitor. Before her eyes, the pressure dropped. Her stare darted to Harvey, a different kind of adrenaline flooding her system. As if making a joint decision, Harvey nodded to Della and unlocked the wheels of the stretcher.

'Send the blood round to theatre,' he said, his voice calm but full of authority. 'Dr Wilton and I are taking him straight to surgery.'

It was the same call Della would have made. There was no time to waste. But as they rushed round to theatre, wheeling the patient with them, what shocked Della most was how good it sounded to hear Harvey automatically refer to them as a team.

CHAPTER SIX

IN THEATRE, HOURS LATER, Harvey sutured the abdominal drain in place and released the clamp, initiating the suction. The drain would remove any residual blood or peritoneal fluid from around the liver laceration, which he and Della had spent the past three hours patching, having slowly and steadily removed the offending tree branch and its splinters. With the exception of two additional nicks in the small intestine, which Della had meticulously repaired, this young man had been incredibly lucky. The internal damage could have been way more extensive and life-threatening.

'Are you happy for me to close?' Harvey asked Della, his back stiff from standing in the OR for so many hours.

Instead of the afternoon off they'd planned, they'd worked together on the complex surgery. Harvey was grateful for the second pair of eyes when it came to the areas of haemorrhage and the fragments of the broken branch they'd found in the man's abdominal cavity. He and Della worked together as if they'd been doing it for years, leaving all of their petty arguments behind, although not their sexual chemistry. Who'd have thought they could get along so well?

Della shifted a retractor, taking one last look at the repaired liver contusion. She wasn't going to be satisfied until she'd checked for herself, and Harvey respected her for that. As a consultant, he'd do the same. Della was an astute and thorough surgeon who didn't allow Harvey's slight seniority in years to deter her from making suggestions or questioning his technique.

'Looks as good as we can expect,' she said finally, her eyes meeting his over the top of her mask.

Harvey nodded in agreement and reached for a needle to close the abdominal wall layers one by one. 'Right, let's close him up. He's certainly not out of the woods yet, but we've done the best we can.' The biggest risk for the patient now that they'd stopped the bleeding was a postoperative complication, especially an infection. Hopefully the cocktail of IV antibiotics Della had started would help, but the young man's recovery would need to be closely monitored.

'I hear they've admitted three more casualties,' Della said, reaching for a second needle to help him close up the laparotomy wound. 'One head injury and two with multiple limb fractures who have been picked up by our orthopaedic colleagues.' She started her sutures at the other end of the vertical surgical incision so they would meet in the middle.

'Busy day,' Harvey agreed, glancing her way. 'We certainly had our hands full with this case. I'm grateful you were here.'

Before Fiji, he'd thought he'd known Della pretty well, but working so closely with her, not to mention their physical connection, was forcing him to take a second and third and fourth look. It was as if he was finally, after all this time, seeing the *real* Della, not the woman he'd spent twenty years avoiding looking at too closely in an attempt to manage his attraction. And it was freaking him out. Especially when she'd all but propositioned him this morning to continue their holiday fling until it was time to go home. Not that he'd needed any persuading.

'No,' she countered, flicking him a challenging look, 'I'm grateful *you* were here.'

Under his mask, Harvey grinned. Just because they'd slept together again, just because they'd agreed on a brief, physical fling, didn't mean their rivalry was completely over. And a part of him wouldn't have it any other way. He'd never felt bored in Della's stimulating, often challenging, company.

He dragged in a breath, his movements with the suture needle and forceps automatic. Now that their patient was stable and out of immediate danger, his mind wandered back to more pleasurable thoughts. There was no point trying to pretend that he was in control of their sexual chemistry, not here where they couldn't walk away from each other as they normally would. Having spent last night reacquainting himself with Della's body, Harvey would be fooling himself if he thought he'd be able to resist her while they were trapped together in Fiji. And as she'd said, a holiday fling was pretty harmless. They knew each other well. They were each invested in a future where they would see each other socially. They understood that when it came to relationships, they were complete opposites: she wanted one and he didn't. But a niggle of caution lodged in his brain. He didn't want to hurt Della. But she knew what she wanted, and for now, it was him; he'd be stupid to pass that up.

'But more compliments, Dr Ward,' Della said when

he'd remained silent for a while. 'Careful, Harvey. There must be something in the Fijian water.' She glanced his way with that playful glint in her eyes.

Harvey chuckled, relieved that the events of last night, first their row and then spending the night together, hadn't affected their relatively new working relationship. That they could respect each other professionally after he'd been appointed to the Melbourne job gave him an enormous amount of satisfaction.

'You'll have my head swelling,' she went on, her movements as practiced as his as they sutured the wound. 'As you know, the Wiltons are such a high-achieving family, it's hard to feel as if you've distinguished yourself.'

Harvey looked up, her comment giving him pause, as if he should have realised she had self-doubts, as if they'd spent twenty years misunderstanding each other. He'd never considered it before, but it must have been hard for her, growing up the youngest in a family of medics.

'But you *have* distinguished yourself,' he pointed out. Was that why Della always seemed to have something to prove? Harvey could relate to that. For a while, during his teens, he'd been determined to show his absent mother what she'd given up on, a part of him striving to be a son of whom she could be proud, as if he'd hoped she'd want to renew their relationship. But the phone had stayed silent. He'd worked hard at school, earned a place at medical school, and become a leading surgeon in one of Australia's top hospitals, but some days, when his mind wandered to his mother, he still felt…inadequate.

'There's no question,' he added, dragging his thoughts from his own upbringing.

She shrugged. 'I guess. Although growing up in Brody's

shadow, nothing I achieved was ever that extraordinary. And then, along came *you*.'

'Me?' Harvey tied off his last suture and cut the ends, his discomfort building.

Della looked up and nodded. 'Yes, *you*.' Her voice was playful, but he sensed she was about to offer information he hadn't known. 'I was just about to leave home for med school,' she continued, 'when Brody brought you home for the weekend that first time. Remember?'

'I remember I upset you with some immature comment about your boyfriend.' If she'd doubted her abilities back then, could that explain her sensitivity to criticism, especially when it had come from some guy she'd never met before?

Della ignored his reference and went on. 'You and Brody had just qualified, just started work as *real* doctors, and you were both insufferable. Strutting around, patronising me with warnings of how hard med school was, teasing me because I was moping over—' She froze. 'Oh, I can't even remember his name…'

'Oliver,' Harvey said, shame and regret hot in his veins as he recalled that weekend when he and Della had made such bad first impressions on each other and the part he'd played.

'Of course, Brody is such a great guy,' she continued as if he hadn't interjected, '*and* he's my brother, so I couldn't hate him for being better than me at everything. But you… You were fair game, I'm afraid.'

Harvey tried to find the humour in the story, but instead, his protective urges for Della fired. 'No wonder we hit it off badly,' he said. It shouldn't matter. The past was in the past, and they were just having sex. But the idea that she'd struggled to believe in herself among her competitive family, fearing she was second best to Brody, the idea of Della displacing her resentment for Brody onto Harvey, left him strangely flat.

Having closed the peritoneum and abdominal muscles, Harvey reached for a staple gun to close the skin. 'You know, I'm not sure if the appointment panel at Melbourne told you this, but you came very close to getting the job they offered me.'

Della stilled. Her eyes met his, full of questions. 'I appreciate you telling me that, Harvey, but I'm a big girl. I can live with second place, and I think they appointed the most experienced candidate at the time.'

Della's confidence in her abilities was attractive, but it was suddenly important to him that she knew of his regard. 'Credit where credit is due,' he said as he placed the final staple and reached for a dressing to cover the wound. 'Surgery is a competitive field. We're all vying for the same positions. Just because I got that job doesn't make me a better surgeon.' With the operation complete, Harvey gave the nod to the anaesthetist to wake the patient before stepping away and removing his mask and gloves.

'I know that—I'm heaps better than you,' she teased as they tossed their surgical gowns in the dirty laundry hamper.

'Well, I wouldn't go that far,' Harvey said as they left theatre to wash up. It was good to have their light-hearted banter back, but the more time he spent with Della, the more he realised that he hadn't really known her before, and he couldn't help but feel he'd missed out.

'You don't have to worry about me, you know,' she said, pausing at the sinks and turning on the taps to wash her hands. 'Despite the fuss I made over your job being rightfully mine, my ego wasn't really dented.' She looked up, met his stare. 'I was just in a bad place at the time, with the divorce. I needed a win. Any win. There's nothing better equipped to make you feel like a big fat failure than a divorce, trust me.'

Harvey reached for a wad of paper towels to dry his hands, a little lost for words that she'd confided in him. He was out of his depth with relationship advice, but he hated the idea that Della blamed herself for her marital breakdown. Harvey didn't know the details, but he was certain it wasn't Della's fault.

'Why would *you* be the failure?' he asked, defensive on her behalf.

'Oh, you know, because I should have seen it coming.' Della switched off the taps and yanked some towels from the dispenser.

Harvey struggled to find the right words. Della had never opened up to him before. 'Do you…want to grab a beer at Savu's?' he asked, wishing they were anywhere but at work so he could touch her, steal the kiss he'd waited all day for, make her smile. 'I'm happy to listen if you want to vent, although, as you know, relationships aren't my strong point.'

He didn't want to put his foot in it again. He watched doubt flit over her expression. He could understand that if she'd grown up feeling second best to Brody, the fact that she was now divorced, whereas her brother was happily married and a dad, might heighten her sense of failure.

'Don't worry, Harvey. There's no relationship to advise on. It's over. Forgotten.' She tossed paper towels in the bin and faced him with a brave face. 'I'm well shot of a man who, by the time we split up, had pretty much convinced me that his career was more important than mine, just because I wanted us to have a family.'

'What?' Harvey scowled, his flare of anger on Della's behalf hot and sharp. 'That's ridiculous.'

She shrugged, looking embarrassed. 'I know relationships are about compromise, but by the end, I felt as if he'd used my career as an excuse to put off talking about us starting a family, as if I couldn't possibly have both. As if I had to make a choice, a family or a career, but why should I? *He* didn't have to. *Brody* didn't have to. *You* wouldn't have to.'

'Why indeed?' Harvey frowned, shocked by the ferocity of his empathy. Had her doubts of being overshadowed by Brody bled into her marriage? Had smart and caring Della settled somehow for her ex's excuses? It was none of Harvey's business, but Della deserved so much better. She deserved someone who would raise her up, not tear her down. She deserved whatever white picket fence dream she chose.

They passed through a door and paused outside their respective changing rooms. It was after hours, their surgery clearly the last one of the day. The place felt deserted. Because it had been too long since they'd kissed, at least nine hours, not that he was counting, Harvey pressed his lips to hers, scooping his arm around her waist. She sighed, gripped his arms and returned his kiss. His thoughts silenced, his body relaxing. Normally he kept people at arm's length, but with Della, because he knew her so well, because she was a big part of his life, because she'd opened up to him, he couldn't help but feel invested.

Before things turned too heated, Harvey pulled back. 'I know we haven't always seen eye to eye over stupid things,' he said, cupping her face, his thumb gliding over her cheekbone, 'but for the record, I think you're amazing.'

He needed to shut up. He was straying out of his comfort zone, but he cared.

'Thanks.' She blinked, clearly touched by his uncharacteristic praise. 'Another compliment. Aren't you scared by the potency of the water?' She smiled, playful, and his heart thumped erratically.

He *was* scared, but not of the water. The real Della, the one he couldn't escape here, the one he was uncovering like an archaeologist exposes a dig, was addictive. It was as if last night had broken some sort of internal restraint. He couldn't seem to keep his hands off her or stop thinking about her and the new things he'd learned.

'I guess you're not so bad yourself,' she said. 'But if we can't trust the water, perhaps we should go for that beer. I'm parched over here.' She was returning to humour as if she could sense the shaky ground on which he was standing and wanted to toss him a lifeline, or perhaps she was also wary of exposing too much. After all, this was about sex.

'Right. Savu's it is.' Harvey released her reluctantly. 'I'll meet you back here in five minutes.'

They parted ways, ducking into their respective changing rooms with matching goofy grins. Harvey removed his scrubs and headed for the shower, using the time to straighten his head. Just because he knew Della well, understood her dreams, had begun to see glimpses into her fears and regrets, didn't mean he could be her confidant. He'd been alone so long, he wasn't even sure he was capable of having more than a casual good time. He certainly knew nothing about the kind of lifelong commitment Della wanted.

Next time she looked sad over her failed marriage or compared herself to Brody, he would do well to remember that not only was he ill-qualified to give relationship advice, but he couldn't be responsible for her happiness. As she'd pointed out, when it came to a man like him, Della was smart enough to have zero expectations.

CHAPTER SEVEN

THE FOLLOWING AFTERNOON, sitting at the front of the two-person kayak with Harvey behind, Della sliced her paddle through the clear sapphire-blue water, a sense of relaxed contentment flooding her system. Maybe it was the warm sun on her back or the salt in her drying hair after their swim. Maybe it was the wonders of the coral reef marine life, the clownfish and the butterflyfish they'd seen while snorkelling. Maybe it was the thrill of beating Harvey back to the kayak in a swimming race and the steamy victory kiss she'd claimed when he'd finally caught up.

Della glanced over her shoulder and caught Harvey's eye. A goofy smile tugged at her cheeks. Maybe it was all those things combined with extreme sexual satisfaction.

'It's so beautiful here,' she said, steering the kayak back across the lagoon towards the white sandy beach of Tokuma Island, a picture-perfect tropical oasis accessible by water taxi from the main island and home to an adults-only holiday resort.

'Hmm,' he agreed, his superior strength propelling the kayak forward. 'Better late than never.'

Della nodded, a small part of her wishing they'd spent their postponed afternoon off in bed. She couldn't seem to get enough of Harvey Ward. The minute he'd arrived to pick her up for their island adventure that morning, she'd dragged him inside her bungalow and kissed him senseless. One thing had rapidly led to another. They hadn't even made it to bedroom this time, simply collapsed onto the sofa, tugging frenziedly at each other's clothes.

'I've had the best afternoon,' Della said, sighing happily as she recalled burying her face against the side of Harvey's neck and crying out her orgasm while Harvey had groaned, crushing her in his arms as he climaxed. Was there any better way to relax than sun, sea and sex? But no matter how hard she tried to compartmentalise their physical relationship, she couldn't help but enjoy Harvey's company—his dry sense of humour, his geeky encyclopaedic knowledge of most subjects, the playful challenge he brought to everything like a dash of spice, keeping life interesting.

Reminding herself to also embrace caution—she couldn't get carried away and forget that he was still the same old Harvey—Della steered the kayak into the shallows. They climbed off and tugged it up onto the sand near the rental place—a palm-roofed shack filled with paddles and snorkel gear. They returned the masks and snorkels to the *used* bin and headed up the beach for the shade of one of the palm leaf umbrellas dotting the shoreline.

At her side, Harvey took Della's hand. She smiled over at him, the breath catching in her chest. She'd been nervous about spending too much time with him, but Fiji Harvey seemed like a completely different man to his Australian counterpart. He was fun and caring, and she had to constantly remind herself that he'd never actually been a boyfriend. His romantic gestures were merely a pretty irresistible form of sexual foreplay.

'I brought some snacks,' Harvey said as they sat on the warm sand. He opened his small backpack to reveal some crackers, a pack of nuts and two apples. 'We need to keep our energy up.' He winked, his suggestive smile sending Della's body molten.

'See, no matter how hard you try to hide it, you *are* a good guy,' she teased, opening the roasted almonds and popping one into her mouth, touched by his thoughtfulness.

'It's true.' Harvey shrugged and took a giant bite from one of the apples. 'That must be why Brody and Amy have asked me to be Jack's mentor for his naming day. I wasn't sure if they'd told you yet.'

He watched her carefully. Obviously *he knew* that Della had also been asked to mentor Jack, the equivalent of a godparent. Della nodded, not in the slightest bit surprised by Brody and Amy's choice. Harvey was Brody's best friend. Of course he would ask him to be there for his only son. But that meant, like it or not, she'd definitely see him again in three weeks' time. By then, their holiday fling would be a distant memory, although it would be hard to forget days like today, when they'd not only had great sex but also had fun and laughed together, making brand-new memories.

'I can't wait for Jack's naming day,' Della said, taking a long drink from her water bottle. 'As his aunt and his mentor, I'll have two excuses for cuddles. Don't tell my brother, but I might even steal him and smuggle him back to New Zealand.' She laughed, but a niggle formed a knot in her chest. She was happy for Brody and Amy, but newly divorced, it had been hard to hear their pregnancy news and not feel a massive pang of longing, as if yet again she was being left behind.

'I'm looking forward to it, too,' Harvey said with an easy smile combined with that hungry stare of his.

'Really?' she asked, trying to picture Harvey holding her baby nephew, who was coming up to six months old. Jack had one bottom tooth and an adorably gummy smile. 'You've never struck me as the kids type.'

Harvey glanced her way, his expression unreadable. 'I like kids just fine. Small, cute humans—what's not to love?'

Della's pulse pounded with excitement as she watched him polish off the rest of the apple. There was something sexy about the way Harvey ate. Of course, there was something sexy about his every move, but she'd never have guessed he'd be comfortable around kids. But thinking about Jack's naming day left her wondering if she and Harvey could successfully ignore their fling once it was over, as they had last time. The idea that they'd revert to bickering strangers doing their best to ignore each other left her unsettled. She didn't want that. Maybe they'd finally become friends once this sexual chemistry had run its course?

She watched a droplet of water trail a path down his toned and golden abs. Nope, having Harvey as a friend seemed unlikely. Or would they still hook up every now and then, before Della moved on to a new relationship?

'Contrary to what some people believe,' he said, distracting her from how exactly their relationship would work in the future, 'I even possess a heart.' He shot her a teasing glance, and stowed the apple core in a paper bag.

Guilt left her flushed. 'I guess we didn't really know each other very well before Fiji,' she said, lying down beside him on the sand, where he was propped up on his elbows. She rested one hand on his chest, brushing at the grains of golden sand that glinted on his skin.

'I guess we didn't,' he said, lying back and pillowing one bent arm under his head. 'I'm glad we finally got the chance to know each other better.' His other hand came to rest on hers, his intense stare shifting over her face.

Della's belly fluttered as if he'd hungrily scoured every inch of her bikini-clad body. She recognised that look, and his touch, no matter how innocent, never failed to turn her on.

'You know,' he said, falling serious, 'I *did* have a relationship once, a girlfriend, before I met you and Brody. I wanted you to know, because...you know, relationships aren't easy, for anyone.'

Della stiffened, gaped, completely at a loss for what to say. Her fingers stilled in his dark chest hair, the rapid thud of his heart under her palm telling her this was hard for him to confess. And was he reassuring her again because she'd told him how her divorce had made her feel like a failure? But Harvey...a girlfriend? He was *Harvey*. Never short of offers but always alone at couple times— Christmas, birthday celebrations, holidays.

'Did you love her?' she asked finally, her raging curiosity an uncomfortable gnawing in the pit of her stomach. Was that what he'd meant when he'd said being vulnerable with another person was a *brave gamble*? Had Harvey had his heart broken and subsequently turned his back on commitment? How had she never known this about him? And why should it matter? She wasn't jealous. It was just that the more time she and Harvey spent together, she realised that she didn't really know him at all.

As if he regretted the impulse to share this with her, Harvey sat up, rested his arms on his bent knees and looked out to sea. 'I don't know…maybe.'

Well, that was vague. The easy, laid-back vibe they'd enjoyed all afternoon while they'd swum and snorkelled the reef departed. That jealousy she'd denied a moment ago slid through Della's veins like fire. Harvey in love? A secret relationship he'd kept from her. Did Brody know?

'What happened?' Della softly asked, scared to pry but even more scared to miss this opportunity to know him better, because in light of his revelation, they seemed like strangers again. 'Did she break your heart?' Was that why he was slow to admit he'd loved this girl? Was that why he'd avoided relationships all these years? It seemed like an extreme reaction, but she didn't want to judge.

'Kind of…' He sighed, keeping his back turned.

'Well, I can understand why you'd be reluctant to confide in me,' Della said. 'After the way I've judged you in the past. If it's any consolation, I regret that now.' Della lay stiffly on the sand, shame holding her tongue. She'd assumed that he was happy with casual sex, but now it seemed that the reality might be much more complex. He *had* been in a relationship once. He'd probably loved someone and had his heart broken. Brody was right— Harvey *did* possess hidden depths.

'It's not that,' he said, turning to face her, his expression stoic. 'It's just hard to talk about. She died in a car collision aged twenty-two. She was a medical student like me. Her name was Alice.'

Della sat up, covered her shocked gasp with her hand,

her heart twisting painfully at the tragic news. 'I'm so sorry, Harvey. I had no idea.'

'It was a long time ago.' Harvey shrugged, returned his gaze to the sea. 'Brody knew that I didn't like to talk about it. I know he's a know-it-all as a brother, but as a friend, he's very loyal.'

Della's mind reeled. She understood that Brody would keep Harvey's secret, but she wished she'd known this vital piece of information sooner. In context, it painted tortured Harvey in a whole new light. He must have really loved this girl. Were heartache and grief the reasons a younger Harvey, the man she'd first met and taken an instant dislike to in a love-hate kind of way, had played the field? Had loving and losing Alice had a profound effect on him, so he avoided further pain by avoiding commitment?

Della swallowed, her throat burning with regret and jealousy. 'Is Alice the reason that you don't date?' she asked in barely a whisper, some part of her needing to know if he was still in love with this woman. Still grieving. Still heartbroken.

'It's not that cut and dried,' he said, keeping his back to her. 'I didn't wake up the next day and make a conscious decision that I was done with relationships for good. It just kind of happened that way.' His shoulders tensed. 'We'd been together a couple of years,' he continued, his voice tight. 'And although it probably wouldn't have lasted, I was devastated to lose her like that, so... suddenly. So pointlessly.'

'Of course you were. Who wouldn't be?' Della reached out and placed her hand between his shoulder blades. Yes, their relationship was about sex, and this Harvey, a complex man hiding a vulnerable side, was a stranger to her, but she couldn't help but comfort him the way he'd tried to do for her at Savu's last night after she'd admitted details of her divorce.

But why wouldn't it have lasted? She desperately wanted to ask, but maybe she'd pried enough. Instead, she pressed her lips to his sun-warmed shoulder, her eyes stinging with emotion. Everything she'd assumed about this man had shattered like glass. He wasn't arrogant and competitive; he was dedicated and driven. He wasn't carefree and single; he was protecting himself. He wasn't two-dimensional; he was complex.

'I guess when the shock and grief faded,' he went on, 'it seemed easier, less effort, to keep my relationships superficial. No need to tell a one-night stand about your sad past. I didn't want to talk about it anyway, even if someone had asked.'

Della caressed his shoulder, too emotional to say anything. Why hadn't *she* asked? Instead, she'd taken him at face value, ridiculed his choices and used him for sex. Twice.

'I focussed on work,' he said, shooting her a wry smile. 'Before I knew it, one year had turned into another and another. By the time five years had gone by, I'd developed casual dating habits—keeping it light and impersonal, having a good time and moving on—that didn't seem to have any downside.' He glanced over his shoulder. 'You know that saying—"if it's not broken, don't fix it"?'

Della nodded in understanding.

'Well, that encompassed my personal life.' He shifted, lay back down on his side, pulling Della down too. 'I guess I just never found a good enough reason to change,' he said, although Della wondered if he might be holding something more back.

He propped his head on one hand, and she mirrored his position so they faced each other in the shade of the umbrella. 'Because relationships are risky,' she said flatly, knowing all about the pitfalls of loving someone and having your heart broken. But whereas Della hoped to find love again in the future, Harvey had found the perfect solution to protect his heart—staying single. He'd never met a woman it was worth risking the status quo for, or he just didn't see that anything was lacking in his personal life, or he was happy with the sacrifice if it meant avoiding pain.

'Don't you ever get lonely?' she asked cautiously, looking down at their clasped hands where his thumb slid against her skin, raising goose bumps on her arm. She doubted she could do what Harvey had done, stay alone all these years. She loved being part of a couple, having someone to share things with, someone who just understood you. Until it went wrong...

'How can I be lonely surrounded by Wiltons?' he said with a small smile, distancing himself from the question and the heavy turn in the conversation.

Della couldn't blame him for putting up emotional barriers. She'd done the same last night when he asked about Ethan.

'So you see,' he said, a twinkle of humour coming into his eyes, 'I'm not heartless. I'm just stuck in my ways. Lazy.'

Della entwined her fingers with his, desperate to ask all the questions building inside. By avoiding long-term relationships, he was keeping himself safe, yes, but wasn't he also missing out on connection, on knowing someone on a deep level as much as they knew him?

'Lazy or scared?' she asked, looking up. She could fully relate to the latter. Putting herself back out there in search of a relationship, of the right man, often seemed too monumental to contemplate, but unlike Harvey, she didn't want to be alone forever.

'You're probably right,' he said. 'Although my explanation puts me in a better light.' As if he wanted to draw a line under the topic, Harvey leaned close and pressed his lips to hers, the heated kiss almost enough of a distraction to end the conversation.

His hand rested on her waist, his tongue sliding against hers. Della sighed, turned on by his touch but still reeling from everything she'd learned about him in the past few days. It was as if she hadn't known the real Harvey at all, as if she'd filed him away in a mislabelled box to keep herself safe from her feelings, and now she needed to re-examine them in the cold light of day. No, there were no feelings beyond attraction and respect. Feelings had no place in their fling.

Pulling back, she rested her forehead against his, breathing hard. 'I understand the fear, you know, the emotional gamble of being vulnerable with another person. Why do you think I haven't bothered with dating since the divorce? I've had my fingers burned, and I'm in no rush to go through that again. It's as if my instincts, my judgement took a massive hit.' That part of her that hadn't seen her marital problems coming was terrified to let another person close, terrified to get it wrong, again. Although her time for meeting *the one*, for falling in love and starting a family, was running out. She'd be forty in two and half years.

'I can understand that.' His searching stare flicked between her eyes, so Della wanted to hide behind her sunglasses. He cupped her face. 'But you deserve to be happy. You deserve to have it all, Della, if that's what you want.'

Della nodded, her throat hot and achy. To be seen for the first time since her divorce, and by Harvey of all people… She *did* want it all, but having what she wanted wasn't straightforward.

'Knowing what you want is the easy part,' she said with a sad laugh, looking down at their clasped hands to hide her eyes from him. 'It's finding someone who wants the same as you that's tricky. I've already got that wrong once.' She didn't want to think about her ex, not lying here hand in hand with Harvey, when they were finally sharing something personal, when she felt so close to him. But now that she knew his reason for avoiding relationships, their differences were more obvious than ever. It wasn't that Harvey wanted to be single. It was that he didn't ever want the risk of a relationship, and to eternally romantic and hopeful Della, that was the most depressing thing she'd heard for a long time.

'It will happen,' Harvey said, an encouraging smile in his eyes. 'You have everything going for you—a great career, an awesome personality, this sexy body…' His smiled stretched, but then he sobered. 'Just don't settle for less than you deserve, okay?'

Della nodded, confused that Harvey, of all people, understood her so well. Had she compromised too much and settled with Ethan? Had she, over time, allowed her ex's dreams to eclipse and squash her own? It hadn't felt that way at the time, but by then end of their marriage, he'd changed. He'd sold her a fairy tale and rewritten the happy ending.

'You deserve to be happy too,' she said tentatively, too scared to know if he was still in love with Alice. 'What does that look like for you? Being alone forever?' Her pulse pounded so hard, she feared he might feel it in her fingers. This degree of emotional intimacy was uncharted territory for them.

'I don't think about forever.' He shrugged, his stare untroubled. 'I just know that right now, my life is good. I'm in control. Why would I mess with that?'

'Ah…the control freak again,' Della said, trying to make light of it even as her heart sank. She told herself she was disappointed for Harvey, because surely everyone wanted to be in love? To share their life with someone? To feel deeply connected to another human being? But maybe for Harvey, control of his emotions was more valuable. And a part of her could understand.

'Don't feel sorry for me,' he said, tugging on her hand and steering them back to playful territory. 'I do all right with ladies, as you know.' He winked, drew her close, captured her lips in another searing kiss that fogged her mind and silenced all her questions.

Bewildered by what she'd learned, Della surrendered to his kiss, her lips parting, their tongues gliding. There was no point stressing Harvey's choices. The two of them were there to have a good time, not to build a relationship, even a friendship. If nineteen years of casual sex hadn't helped him get over Alice, what chance did Della have in two weeks? He wasn't hers. He wasn't anyone's. If she became distracted by the real Harvey, the man she was coming to understand more deeply every day, she might forget to focus on their physical relationship. She might forget how they still wanted different things, and likely always would.

She gripped his biceps and lost herself, her body sliding closer to his until her breasts grazed his bare chest and their thighs touched. As their kisses built in intensity, she grew aware that she was only wearing a bikini and Harvey board shorts. They were on a public beach on an island popular with snorkellers. They might be in paradise, but they weren't alone.

Breaking away, she calmed her excited breathing. 'We should, um, head back. The last water taxi is at seven.'

Harvey nodded, sliding his legs from the tangle of hers with a wince. 'Just give me a second.'

She smiled, glancing at the bulge in his shorts. When he was ready, they gathered up their belongings and walked hand in hand towards the resort and the dock for the water taxi. As she sat snuggled into him on the boat, her back to his front and his arms around her waist, Della was stunned by how little she'd known Harvey before and how much they had in common beyond their jobs. This man, the dedicated doctor protecting his vulnerable heart, was way more dangerous to her than the carefree ladies' man she'd easily dismissed for close to twenty years.

But Della still wanted the future she'd been denied— love, marriage, a family. And when she finally overcame her fear, when she was finally ready to risk her heart again, she couldn't afford to make another mistake. Next time she fell in love, she needed to get it right.

CHAPTER EIGHT

THE NEXT DAY in the ED was hectic. Harvey and Della had no planned operations, so they'd split up to help the local doctors with the surgical admissions. Harvey had just finished seeing a six-year-old there on holiday with suspected appendicitis when a text came through from Della.

I have a patient who needs a second opinion if you're free.

Harvey washed his hands, his eagerness to reunite with Della leaving him jittery. Yesterday had been a big day. After their kayaking adventure at Tokuma Island, after he'd opened up to her about Alice's death and she'd hinted again at her regrets over her marriage, she'd spent the night at his bungalow. They'd wordlessly showered together, lazily washing the sand and salt from each other's body before falling into bed. They hadn't talked about their pasts again. It was as if they were each processing what they'd learned. The trouble was that by spending so much time with her, by discovering new things about Della, by constantly needing to touch her, Harvey was struggling to keep his emotions in check. He felt out of control, and that was a huge concern. Her words from the day before looped in his mind.

You deserve to be happy too... What does that look like for you? Being alone forever?

Distracted anew by the power of that question, Harvey went in search of Della. He'd never seriously considered it before, but now that she'd raised the idea, now that it was out there in his consciousness, he couldn't seem to put it out of his mind. Nor did he know the answer. Maybe he shouldn't have let Della in yesterday, but he'd wanted her to know that most people had relationship regrets, that she wasn't alone.

Harvey found Della in a nearby bay with an anxious-looking couple in their thirties. As always, his pulse banged at the sight of her, his fingers restless to touch her soft, sun-kissed skin, his lips eager for those passionate kisses that always escalated out of their control.

'Dr Ward,' Della said, her expression both apologetic and relieved. 'Thanks for coming. Mr and Mrs Beaumont would like a second opinion, and I told them you're Melbourne's top trauma surgeon.' Her stare carried questions, as if checking he was okay after his confession yesterday. But he'd rather she look at him with desire than pity.

'Only because they were too stupid to appoint you, Dr Wilton.' Harvey smiled at the patient, Mr Beaumont, who was lying on the stretcher, supporting his left arm in a sling.

Della was a compassionate doctor, a talented surgeon and a good listener. She would be a catch for any man. Harvey hated to see the threads of doubt she carried. Yes, she knew what she wanted, but she also felt that she'd compromised too much in her marriage.

'The Beaumonts are here on their honeymoon,' Della told Harvey. 'Mr Beaumont is a fit and healthy thirty-year-old who fell off a jet ski this morning travelling at approximately fifty kilometres per hour. He sustained a mild concussion on hitting the water and has an anterior dislocation of the left shoulder.'

Harvey listened as Della pulled up the shoulder X-ray on the computer, which clearly displayed the dislocation. She angled the screen so the newlyweds could also see the results. Harvey quickly examined the man's arm and then scrutinised the X-ray and read the report, in no doubt of Della's diagnosis. It was a standard case of shoulder dislocation, but some patients needed a second opinion. That didn't mean Harvey was better equipped to treat this patient than Della. He trusted her clinical acumen unreservedly. In fact, he realised with an internal jolt, he trusted her, full stop.

That was why he'd told her about Alice. But when had that change happened…?

'So I'm afraid, as Dr Wilton pointed out,' Harvey said, standing side by side with Della in solidarity, 'you have a dislocated shoulder. I agree with her diagnosis.'

Harvey glanced Della's way, hoping she saw his absolute faith in his stare. But standing close without touching her left him restless to drag her into his arms and chase off all her doubts. The same fiercely protective urges he'd experienced yesterday at the beach when she'd told him about her ex-husband flared anew now. What was going on with him, and how could she make him feel this way when he'd effortlessly avoided it for twenty years?

'The good news,' he added to Mr Beaumont, 'is that there doesn't appear to be any fracture or significant tendon or muscle damage, so you won't need surgery. But I concur one hundred percent with Dr Wilton's clinical assessment and the treatment she's suggested.'

Tearful, Mrs Beaumont dabbed at her eyes with a tissue and gripped her husband's hand on his uninjured side. Harvey could sympathise. Of course the wife would be worried. No one wanted their honeymoon marred by injury, but these things happened when you came off a jet ski at speed. The man was lucky the injuries weren't more serious, particularly the concussion.

'Once we put the shoulder back in place,' Della said, her voice reassuring, 'and once the pain and swelling have gone down, you should make a full recovery. If you're happy for us to proceed, we can quickly pop your shoulder back into the joint. The sooner we do that, the less the risk of surrounding tissue damage. Why don't you two chat about it for a moment.'

Harvey and Della left the bay and moved a short distance away so they wouldn't be overheard.

'Thanks for sticking up for me so heartily back there,' she said, looking up at him with a curious smile, perhaps because in the past, when Brody teased her at family gatherings, Harvey had always kept quiet or joined in. If he'd known back then how Della's feistiness was a shield because she compared herself to Brody, how she felt the need to prove herself, how she considered her divorce in particular a personal failure, he'd have been way more tactful.

'Any time, Della.' Shame for how he'd behaved when he'd been focussed on keeping a lid on his attraction for Della coiled inside him. 'You know it's not personal— some patients just like to question everything.'

'Of course.' Della nodded, a flicker of amusement in her stare. Then she sobered and frowned. 'Are *you* okay?' she asked, glancing around the department to make sure they were alone. 'You know...after yesterday. You were gone when I got out of the shower.'

'I wanted to get in a run before work,' he said, shaking off the unfamiliar swarm of emotions that yesterday's confessions, both his and hers, had churned up. 'But I'm fantastic,' he said, staring intently. 'I had a great sleep and woke up feeling...energised.' He'd kissed her awake, as if reaching for her naked body next to him had become the most natural thing in the world, and he wanted her to look at him as she had when he'd pushed inside her and rode them both to orgasm. Would he still reach for her back in Melbourne? Would he crave the scent of Della's perfume on his pillow? Would he acclimatise to having an empty bed again? The idea was mildly depressing...

Della flushed and shot him a censorious look. 'I remember,' she said. 'No need to brag.'

Harvey reined in his smug smile. 'Shall I leave this to you?' he asked about the shoulder dislocation. 'You don't need me.' Although he'd somehow grown used to them working together. They made a great team. Another thing he'd have to get used to when he returned to Australia.

Della shrugged, her ego clearly undamaged. 'I think the wife just expected a prescription for some painkillers and to be sent on their way.'

Harvey bit his tongue, mildly insulted on Della's behalf that her skills had been questioned. A junior doctor could reduce a shoulder dislocation, whereas Della was an experienced consultant trauma surgeon.

'If you have a moment,' she went on, 'I could use your

assistance. I prefer Matsen's traction to reduce a shoulder dislocation, and it's a two-person job.'

'Really? Matsen's?' Harvey asked about her choice of technique mainly because he enjoyed evoking the sparks of challenge in her eyes.

'Yes, Matsen's.' She smiled a mocking smile, clearly onto him and in no way intimidated.

'You don't use the Milch manoeuvre?' he pressed, questioning her to bring out the barely disguised amusement in her stare. 'That's what *I* prefer...' These days, since they were getting along so much better, they weren't sparring as much. Part of him missed it, and maybe Della did, too.

'Well, it doesn't surprise me that we're different,' she said calmly. 'But my technique is better. And it's *my* patient.'

Harvey grinned, glad to see Della wouldn't let him get away with anything, despite the fact that she might be starting to trust him too. After all, she had opened up about her ex. 'Then it's your call,' he said, happily yielding.

'Good. Matsen's it is.' She shot him a victorious look. 'Come on. That shoulder isn't going to right itself. I'm sure the Beaumonts want to get back to their honeymoon.'

Dutifully, Harvey followed her back to the bedside. A week ago, when Della and he only knew the superficial things about each other, they might have more fiercely argued the point on whose technique was better, although there were many. But it didn't matter. They both knew the important thing was to quickly put the head of the humerus back into the joint.

After some time to consider, the patient was happy to

proceed with the treatment. With Mr Beaumont lying on his back and the bed lowered, Della and Harvey took up their positions opposite each other, Della taking hold of the injured arm and Harvey standing next to the man's opposite shoulder. Harvey gripped the ends of a sheet passed around the man's chest and under his affected armpit, while Della held his dislocated arm in position, bent to ninety degrees at the elbow.

'Ready?' she asked the patient, who nodded and then closed his eyes, squeezing his wife's hand.

Della held Harvey's eye contact, silently mouthing *one, two, three* so they were in sync. She leaned back, applying traction to the patient's bent arm, while Harvey pulled on the sheet, applying counter-traction in the opposite direction. With a slight pop, the dislocation reduced, and the patient released a long sigh of relief.

Della flashed Harvey a grateful and triumphant smile that made him want to kiss the living daylights out of her. Instead, he beamed. 'Good old Matsen's. Worked like a charm.'

Della carefully hid her smile, clearly trying to stay professional in front of the patient. They thought differently on many subjects, but when it mattered, they'd proved time and again this week that they could compromise. Would they remember that when they saw each other in the future, or would they revert to bickering over nothing? Had this fling in Fiji forever altered their relationship? Harvey hoped so. He didn't want to go backwards where Della was concerned. Did that mean he wanted to be her friend? *Friends* seemed inadequate after everything they'd shared. But he couldn't seriously be thinking they could be more than friends, could he?

'Who's Matsen?' Mrs Beaumont asked, confused, interrupting the disconcerting turn of Harvey's thoughts.

Della flushed and shot Harvey a disapproving glare. 'It's the name of the technique we just used to relocate your husband's shoulder. Dr Ward and I differ on most things, so we'd discussed our preferences outside.'

Funny how those differences of theirs seemed less important here in Fiji. Harvey excused himself to the couple, quietly addressing Della before he left the bedside. 'Don't forget we have that bilateral laparoscopic acromioplasty to get to.' The made-up medical procedure was their secret code for a coffee break.

'I'll be there shortly,' she said with a straight face, turning to the patient with instructions. 'You'll need to wear a sling for the pain, and to help the swelling go down. I'll prescribe you some analgesia for the discomfort, but an ice pack will help too. And needless to say—no more jet-skiing.'

Harvey headed to the break room and flicked on the kettle, the euphoria of working with Della eclipsed by the return of his unsettled thoughts for the future. He made hot drinks, coffee for him and tea for Della, and then crossed the corridor to the deserted doctors' office to check his emails as a distraction, which was where Della found him a few minutes later.

'Thank you for your help back there,' she said, coming into the room. 'And thanks for trusting my technique. I know it's hard for you to take a back seat, control freak that you are.' She pursed her lips playfully, but all Harvey could think about was kissing her. Maybe then he would remember that this was about sex, not friendship or…feelings. Because when it came to relationships, to more than a casual good time, he had no idea what he was doing.

'For you, I'm always happy to take a back seat,' he said, dipping his head closer and dropping his voice in order to distract them both. 'Especially when we're so good together, in and out of work.'

Della laughed, a tiny shudder passing through her body, so he knew she was thinking about last night and this morning, about their near insatiable physical need for each other. Harvey pushed closed the door before drawing her into his arms. 'Is it wrong that I find your bedside manner incredibly sexy?' Without waiting for a response, he pressed his lips to hers, groaning when she speared her fingers through his hair and deepened the kiss.

This was under his control. Feelings had no place in what they were doing. Harvey was most likely having a wobble because he'd opened up to Della about Alice yesterday. Letting someone that close felt...unnatural. But Della had a way of sneaking under his guard.

'It could be considered mildly perverted,' she teased, tugging his lips back to hers.

Harvey gripped her waist and pressed her up against the closed door, pinning her with his hips. 'How can I want you again?' he asked, his lips sliding down the side of her neck. 'I'm seriously concerned for my own health. I feel like that Aussie marsupial mouse, antechinus, that commits reproductive suicide, literally dying from sex-fuelled exhaustion.'

Della laughed, gasped, tilted her head, exposing her neck to his lips. 'Don't be so dramatic. You know very well that the ultraviolet in sunlight increases testosterone levels. You're just holiday horny.'

He laughed and she brought his mouth back to hers, her body writhing restlessly as his hand delved under her blouse to feel bare skin. Thank goodness he wasn't alone. They couldn't seem to keep their hands off each other. Forcing himself to pull back, he rested his forehead against hers. 'I didn't just lure you here for this, you know. I made you a cup of tea.'

'Thank you, but you can lure me anytime.' She kissed him one last time and then pushed him away. 'That being said, we have the entire afternoon of work to get through.' She wiped at his mouth, presumably at the traces of her lip gloss, and straightened her blouse. 'Are you going to Dr Tora's barbecue tonight? We could walk to his place together if you are. It's not far from the hospital, apparently.'

'I'd love to walk with you,' he said, reaching for her hand, his restlessness building now that she was no longer in his arms. Touching her had become a compulsion, one he was trying not to overthink. Their days in Fiji were numbered. With him back in Melbourne and Della returning to Auckland, the necessary break would happen naturally, and Harvey would surely shake off this feeling that, for the first time in twenty years, a relationship that went beyond sex might not be so bad.

'We'd better get back to work,' she said sheepishly. 'The ED is filling up out there.'

Harvey nodded, his hands reluctantly slipping from her waist. 'If I don't see you before, I'll call for you at seven tonight.'

'It's a date.' She smiled, and he felt instantly lighter. She opened the door and ducked out of the office.

Harvey lingered for a few minutes more, trying to

straighten his head. Could he and Della really go back to their former relationship after sharing so much? Could he see her at Jack's naming day and not want her? Could he watch her date and fall in love again without being eaten alive with jealousy?

But what was the alternative? Trying to have more than a physical fling with Della would surely put important areas of his life at risk—his newfound truce with her, his friendship with Brody, his valuable place in the Wilton family. Was he seriously considering taking those risks, not to mention the personal risks to him: that powerlessness he detested so much?

Because if he wasn't careful, if he overstretched and tried to have more than a fling, he might hurt Della and damage his relationships with all of the Wiltons. With those stakes, Harvey had the most to lose.

CHAPTER NINE

LATER THAT EVENING, after a family barbecue at the beautiful beachside home of Dr Tora, Della and Harvey waved goodbye and set off for the stroll back to their hospital accommodation. As soon as they were out of sight of the older man's elegant wooden villa, Harvey reached for Della's hand.

She smiled, shuddered, his touch now familiar but still new enough to affect her entire body with tingles. Because for Della, what had begun as *just sex* was now way more complicated.

'You okay?' he asked, picking up on her strange mood as they headed along the sand. 'You seem a bit quiet.'

'I'm fine—a little tired maybe.' Della faked a big smile, too confused by the way she felt to say more. She'd never in a million years have predicted that her and Harvey's previously strained relationship would turn so harmonious and confusing. Working together, sleeping together, discovering new things about him; it was intense. And now, where Harvey was concerned, she could no longer easily untangle her feelings. She only knew they were dangerous.

'That was a lovely night,' she said to take her mind off the rush of panic. She stepped close, holding on to his arm with her other hand so they could walk side by side along the beach. 'Watching you get thrashed at footy by Dr Tora's grandchildren was a particular highlight for me.'

Harvey smiled, and Della relaxed. She didn't want to drag the evening down with her solemn mood, nor could she explain herself anyway. It wasn't like she could tell Harvey that uncovering his *hidden depths* had changed how she saw him and cracked open the lid on feelings she'd spent years denying. She knew it was ridiculous, but a part of her, the part she was scared to examine too closely, wondered if, in another life, they might have stood a chance of something more than just physical. But Harvey didn't want more.

'That little wiry one kept cheating,' Harvey said, the humour in his dark stare setting off another cascade of longing in Della. 'I caught him literally moving the goalposts more than once.'

Della chuckled, although in truth, the sight of Harvey, playful and sporty, engaging with the group of differing aged kids had made her mouth dry with lust and something else. Fear. Was she at risk of developing real romantic feelings for Harvey?

Her stomach tight with unease, Della clung to the lighter topic. 'I guess that's easily done when the goal is an imaginary line between two coconuts, but well done for being a good sport. I'm not sure Brody would have let them win. He's too competitive.'

And right now, as befuddled as she felt, she really needed Harvey to be rubbish with kids, rubbish at *something*, although if he'd sworn off relationships, he obviously had no burning desire to become a father.

'Speaking of kids,' he said, glancing her way as if he

somehow knew the path her mind had wandered, 'it's Mother's Day tomorrow. Don't forget to message Mrs W.'

Della watched him curiously, her hormones firing once more. Harvey really cared about her mother. Why had she never noticed that before? It was as if, when it came to Harvey, she'd been walking around with her eyes closed.

'If you don't mind,' he added, pulling his phone from his pocket, 'I was going to send her this picture of us.'

Della took a closer look. They were standing together on Dr Tora's veranda with the sea behind them, smiling into the camera, looking tanned and relaxed, Harvey's head tilted in Della's direction.

'Of course not,' Della mumbled, shocked by the contentment she saw shining in her own eyes. Would her mother recognise it? Would Jenny Wilton have awkward questions for them when they were next all together for Jack's naming day? No, she too knew Harvey well enough to know that any sort of relationship would be the last thing on *his* mind. It should be the last thing on Della's mind too, but perhaps this fling had simply proved she was finally ready to move on and start dating again.

Della passed the phone back. Everyone looked happy on holiday, especially if they were also having oodles of awesome sex. Her look of contentment didn't mean anything.

'Do you always wish my mother happy Mother's Day?' she asked, surprised. It just occurred to her that Harvey rarely talked about his own mother. Della knew his parents were divorced, but she'd always assumed his mother must have died.

Harvey shrugged, slipping his phone back into the pocket of his shorts. 'Your parents are like family to me.

Mrs Wilton is the closest thing I have to a mother. She's always been so warm and welcoming. I send her flowers on her birthday, too.' He shot her a smug smile, and Della's pulse fluttered at his thoughtfulness.

'You complete and utter suck-up,' Della said in mock outrage. 'Show up me and Brody, why don't you.' But her rampant curiosity flared into an inferno. 'What happened to *your* mother? I've never heard you talk about her.'

A week ago she wouldn't have dared ask him such a personal question. But she and Harvey had come a long way since that first day in Fiji. Now he was her first thought when she opened her eyes. His appearance brought excitement, not annoyance. With every day that passed, with every new revelation she learned, she felt their deepening emotional connection. Perhaps that was the problem. It was time to go home and leave their holiday and their fling behind... She swallowed that metallic taste of fear. It would be a relief to leave Fiji next week, so she could feel back to normal.

'My parents split up when I was eight,' Harvey said, stiffening slightly at her side. 'She wasn't around much after that.' He kicked at a seashell, sending it skittering along the sand.

Della held her breath, a knot forming under her ribs. Brody often said that Harvey didn't like to rake over the past, but there was obviously more to the story. 'But she's still alive?' Della gently pushed, wondering if his estranged relationship with his mother shaped him. How could it not?

He nodded, keeping his face turned away, his gaze trained on the ocean and the setting sun on the horizon.

'She visited for a while after she left my dad. But soon, her visits dwindled.'

Della's stomach clenched with empathy. Why? Surely she'd want to see her son? 'I'm sorry, Harvey,' she whispered. 'That must have been hard for you and Bill.'

Why had she never asked about his mother before? Why had she never bothered to scratch the surface of this complex man? Out of fear, maybe, because she'd been trying to keep her distance? Falling for twenty-three-year-old Harvey Ward would have been younger Della's stupidest move. If the timing had been right for them both when they'd first met, she suspected that she would have fallen hard.

He shrugged, but now that she knew the real man so much better, Della tensed, instinctively attuned to his vulnerability. 'I was lucky,' he said, almost as if persuading them both. 'I got to live with my dad. He's a great father who always made time for me.'

'I have a lot of respect for Bill,' Della agreed. 'But as a kid, you would have loved both your parents.' She couldn't seem to let this go, as if finally she'd caught a glimpse of the innermost layer of Harvey Ward. The missing piece of the puzzle that would put everything into perspective and maybe help Della untangle her conflicted feelings.

Harvey winced, and Della's heart broke for him. 'I was torn in the beginning,' he said simply, but she felt him stiffen. 'Being happy to stay with my dad felt wrong, as did begging for my mother to take me with her every time she visited and then left again.'

'That's a horrible position to be in.' Della blinked away

the sting in her eyes, grateful for the failing light. 'No kid should feel as if they have to choose a parent.'

What had his mother's repeated abandonment done to intelligent, caring Harvey? He must have felt so confused. Yes, he was close to his father, but that wouldn't wholly make up for his absent mother. No wonder he'd kind of adopted *Mrs W*, as he affectionately called Jenny Wilton, as an honorary mother.

'In the end, my mother made the choice for me.' He turned to face her, a sad, bitter smile touching his lips and his eyes hard. 'By the time I was ten, she'd remarried a man who had two little girls and moved out of state. I didn't really hear from her again after that. She chose her new life, her new stepdaughters, over me.'

Della's chest ached, her sore heart racing. Harvey had grown up feeling rejected by the one woman who was supposed to always be there for him, to love him unconditionally with a mother's special brand of love. Had that abandonment strengthened his reaction to his girlfriend's sudden death, made him the self-confessed loner who didn't believe in commitment and love?

'I wish I'd known this sooner,' Della said, her world rocked by his confession and what it meant. Did he want to be alone forever, or was he, like Della, simply scared to risk his heart again because life had taught him that the women he loved disappeared or let him down, or chose someone else?

This past week, buffeted by revelation after revelation, she'd just about managed to cling to their carefree and casual sexual chemistry. But how could she keep her feelings for Harvey in check, knowing what she now knew? How could she fit him back inside that box where she was safe from the way he made her feel—as if they might actually stand a chance?

'I don't like to talk about it,' he said, his voice gruff. 'It's bad enough to remember how powerless I felt at the time, to admit how many years I spent pushing myself, trying to be a son she could be proud of in the hopes that she'd one day come back for me.'

Della squeezed his hand. 'I understand.' Of course he would feel powerless, never knowing if or when his mother might visit, wondering if he'd done something wrong, grieving and confused. Driven, intelligent Harvey would hate feeling that way. And then history had kind of repeated itself when Alice too was suddenly and definitively ripped from his life. No wonder he chose to keep his relationships superficial after that to avoid the risk of being hurt again. Harvey liked to be in control, and there was nothing worse than love for turning your world upside down.

Della reeled as they walked in silence for a few minutes. But she couldn't stay quiet for long, not when Harvey's pain was palpable. When the real Harvey, scarred and battle-weary, called to her, because they had so much in common. When it would be so easy to fall for the man she was getting to know, but for one giant obstacle: he wasn't the right man because they still wanted different things.

'You know,' she said, gripping his arm, 'you're not powerless now. You said it yourself—your life is good. You're successful and hot and, despite trying to hide it from me for the past nineteen years, a really good guy. *I'm* proud of you, especially given I used to think you were just a jerk.' Della tried to smile, clinging to humour to keep things light, desperate to feel the way she used to feel about him, before they'd come to Fiji. With that Harvey, she'd known exactly what to expect. She'd known she was safe.

Harvey returned Della's smile, dragging her close and pressing a kiss to her forehead. 'I see the need to offer compliments is catching. Maybe we should get off this island before we fall madly in love with each other.'

Della stiffened, his joke falling flat. There was something about it she just couldn't find funny, as if one more revelation, one more day working at his side or night in his arms would push her over the edge towards deep, deep feelings.

'It's not magical water, Harvey.' Retreating to their usual banter, Della forced herself to remember that it had been twenty years since Harvey had so much as thought about a relationship, let alone love. His mother's rejection was as heartbreaking as his girlfriend's death, but whatever his reasons for staying single, it meant that Harvey was seriously inexperienced when it came to commitment. She might like, respect and empathise with him now, but she'd still be a fool to fall for a man with so little relationship history, who only wanted to be in control of his feelings. *She* wanted more, so much more.

'Phew, well, that's a relief,' he said, casting her a playful smile and slinging his arm around her waist, the subject closed.

Della walked at his side on shaky legs, glad to have the conversation back on lighter topics. She *wasn't* stupid. When she was ready to fall in love again, she needed a man who knew what he wanted, whose dreams of commitment and a family matched her own. She wouldn't make the same mistake—falling for the wrong guy—twice.

But later, just before she drifted off to sleep in Harvey's bed, her mind returned to the idea that, with the exception of him being so rusty when it came to relationships and having very good reasons for protecting his heart, Harvey ticked an awful lot of boxes.

CHAPTER TEN

THE NEXT DAY was Sunday. Harvey suggested a walk to Vatuwai Falls, the relatively remote waterfall Dr Tora had recommended to them the day before. They'd spent the past hour walking inland from the nearest village, holding hands when the width of the track through the forest allowed. Of course, with Della wearing her sexy denim cut-off shorts, which made her backside look great, single file also had its advantages.

'There it is,' Della called excitedly over the sound of tumbling water. She shot him an excited smile and rounded the final bend in the forest track ahead of Harvey, disappearing out of sight.

Harvey lengthened his strides to catch up, Della's enthusiasm contagious. But she made everything better, brighter, richer. They laughed together. He slept more soundly with her in his arms. She even made the workday pass quicker. What was he going to do without her back in Australia? And how had she sneaked so close that he'd opened up and told her about his mother?

'I'm going in,' Della said as he joined her at the edge of the water.

The falls were nestled in the shade of the island's lush rainforest, the pool beneath ten feet of cascading water, cool and inviting. And they had the place to themselves. Della dropped her backpack and took off her T-shirt and shorts to reveal her gorgeous bikini-clad body, her stare full of that familiar challenge that boiled his blood. Harvey's mouth, already thirsty from the heat of the day and the physical exertion of the trek from the car, dried further with longing. How could he want her again when they'd had sex at sunrise? How would he ever switch off this ravenous craving? How would he see her in the future and not want her the way he wanted her now?

It was crazy, but since they'd started to get to know each other on a deeper, personal level, since he'd seen her fears and insecurities and felt comfortable to open up to her about his past, he'd started to imagine things. Terrifying things. Things that took the control he loved and snapped it clean in two.

Could Della and he have something more than a sexual fling? Could she ever take him seriously? Could she ever want a man like him? Della dreamed of the whole fairy tale, and he was not only severely rusty when it came to feelings, he was also scared that he might be broken. Maybe it was just the magic of Fiji, the dreamlike bubble away from reality. Perhaps it was that until they'd been forced to spend time together, he hadn't really known the real Della at all, and it was just messing with his head.

'Careful,' he called as she gingerly traversed the rocks at the edge of the pool before stepping into the ankle-deep water. They were at least an hour's walk away from the nearest village and further to proper medical care. If one of them slipped, had an accident out here, they'd be in serious trouble.

'Come on, Harvey; it's lovely.' Della ignored his warning and waded into deeper water, the surface lapping against the tops of her thighs, wetting her coral-pink bikini bottoms. Before his brain could re-engage, she dived under the water and surfaced closer to the plunge pool at the base of the waterfall.

Harvey dropped his backpack next to hers and quickly removed his T-shirt and shoes. He was already wearing board shorts, so he followed Della into the pool, the shock of cool water on his skin a welcome reset to the fire she'd set in his blood. When the water reached his hips, he dived in and swam in swift strokes after Della.

'Keep up,' she said, turning onto her back and laughing.

Della was a strong swimmer—she'd told him it was the only sport Brody wasn't good at, because he didn't have the patience to train—and she loved to throw out challenges. Normally he was happy to accept them. But today, maybe because he'd told her about his mother last night, maybe because he'd been reminded how Della's family was also his, how he needed the Wiltons more than ever what with Bill's diagnosis, he was feeling exposed. Needing to get his hands on her to switch off that part of his brain focussed on reason and problem-solving, the part wondering if they could possibly work in the real world, when Harvey had abandoned the things Della wanted years ago, he powered through the water, catching up to her at the base of the waterfall. Della laughed, tried to get away, splashed him in the face.

She might be a stronger swimmer, but Harvey was faster. He snagged her around the waist, treading water as he dragged her nearly naked body against his, so she was all soft curves and slippery skin, taunting him with the things he couldn't have. Because soon, he'd have to give her up, give this up.

The minute they touched, Della back in his arms where she felt way too right, need roared through his blood. 'You always keep me on my toes, do you know that?' He dipped his mouth to hers, captured her smiling lips and kissed her.

She draped her arms around his shoulders and kissed him back, her lips parting, her tongue sliding against his so his arousal flickered in his shorts. 'Well, just because you like to be in control, we can't have you growing complacent.' Laughing, she wriggled free of his arms and kicked away.

Complacent? How could he ever feel settled around Della? She made him unstable, as if he was spinning at the centre of a whirlwind, caught between opposing emotions— fear that he could never be what she needed and an almost overwhelming desire to let her in anyway. But he'd spent twenty years keeping people, including Della, out.

Needing her touch to dampen some of the panic, Harvey caught her again, gripping her waist. 'No chance to be complacent with you around,' he mumbled against her lips, stealing another kiss. To douse the heat they generated when they touched and to pay Della back for the splash to the face, Harvey kicked his legs, guiding them both under the cascading wall of water. The force and shock of the water hitting their heads broke them apart, gasping.

On the far side of the falls, Della laughed, reached for his shoulders and kissed him playfully. 'You always have to win, don't you?'

'Of course.' He grinned, his stomach hollow. There

was one aspect of his life where he hadn't excelled: relationships. Even if Della wanted more than these two stolen weeks in Fiji, with him of all men, was he capable of giving her more than sex? He didn't want to let her down or cause her pain. She'd been hurt enough in the past, and hurting her would mean disappointing, possibly losing, all the Wiltons. But could he really walk away, knowing that this attraction between them had always been there, knowing that he would see her again and again, knowing that now he had nowhere left to hide? She knew all his shameful secrets.

She kissed him, her tongue surging against his as her legs wrapped around his waist under the water. Her bikini-clad body scalded his skin, driving him from memories to the present. Harvey gripped her waist, his toes touching the rocky bottom of the pool. Behind the waterfall, the sunlight was dappled, and the natural pool of shoulder-high water extended into a cave carved from the rocks of the overhanging cliff. Some primal urge shifted through him, a feeling that they might be the only two people on the planet. Nothing seemed to matter beyond how her touch, her kisses, her saying his name made him feel... invincible.

'Why can't I keep my hands off you?' he groaned, growing harder inside his swim shorts as she dropped her head back, exposing her neck to his kisses.

'I know what you mean.' She gripped his waist tighter with her thighs, her breasts bobbing on the surface of the water, their creamy curves teasing him, as if begging for his touch, his mouth. Harvey cupped one breast, his hand sliding down her bikini top and raising the nipple to his lips.

'Harvey...' She sighed and slipped her fingers through his wet hair, releasing her hold on his waist so she slid a little further down his hips.

The heat of her bathed his erection through his shorts. He was struggling to think again, his only instinct to bury himself inside her and chase the mind-numbing oblivion that was never far away when they touched. If he could focus on this, on pleasure, for just a few more days, surely his perspective would return once he was away from the temptation of Della.

Harvey untied the top of her bikini so the cups fell. He switched sides, his grip on her waist tightening as he laved the other nipple. He looked up. Della was watching him, her eyes heavy with desire.

'I want you all the time,' he said, turning them around and backing up against the rocky ledge at the edge of the pool so he could hold her there with his hips. 'What are we doing to each other?'

'I don't know, but let's not stop yet,' she said, gasping when his hand slid between her legs and inside her bikini bottoms.

He was out of control for her, a rage of hormones and terrifying feelings. Fear gripped his throat. What if this all-consuming need for each other didn't fade once they returned to their respective lives in Australia and New Zealand? What if a part of him always pined for Fiji, for Della? What if seeing her back in the real world brought the nice, neat life he'd constructed for himself crashing down around his head? What if she was the only person who could fix it, but she didn't want him?

Before his thoughts could disappear down that blind-ending tunnel, Della slid her hand between their bodies, inside his shorts, and cupped his erection, massaging him in her tight fist so his mind blanked. Harvey dragged his mouth from hers, the last thread of reason strung taut to the snapping point. 'We don't have a condom.'

'I'm okay without it if you are,' she said, kissing the side of his neck while she continued to stroke him under the water.

Harvey groaned, capturing her lips once more. They trusted each other. Knew each other. Neither of them would put the other at risk. Because he was consumed by desire, because she was looking at him as if he could give her everything she needed, Harvey untied one side of Della's bikini bottoms so the fabric slid away from between her legs.

She braced her arms around his shoulders as she sank a little lower, her stare holding his. 'I want you, Harvey.'

Triumph rocked him. He gripped her waist and pushed inside her, the heat of her fanning the rampant flames in his belly. Could she want him for more than sex? Could he give her what she deserved, what she craved? Commitment? But what if he failed, let her down, ruined things for them and for himself?

'Yes,' she hissed as he filled her, her lips parted on her soft gasp, distracting him from thoughts that had no place in what they'd agreed to: a fling.

He cupped her face, bringing her mouth back to his, pressing his tongue against hers, overtaken by an uncontrollable sense of wildness to focus only on this physical connection they'd found and moulded into something unfamiliar but so meaningful.

'Don't stop,' she said when they parted for air. She spread one arm and clung to the rocky ledge at her back while Harvey gripped her waist under the water, held her close to the rhythmic thrust of his hips.

'You're beautiful. I've never wanted anyone this much,' he choked out, watching arousal darken her eyes. 'You know I've always felt this way about you, don't you, since that first time we met?'

She gasped at his honest declaration, something in her stare telling him she too had denied their attraction. But there was no point hiding it. She made him crazy and always had, this possibility there between them since the start, as if waiting for the time to be right. But was *right* enough? As soon as Della was ready to date, she'd be looking for *the one*. Whereas Harvey was so far behind when it came to relationships, he might never catch up. They might never be on the same page. What if he tried and failed?

Because he didn't want to think about where that would leave him once they returned to normality, Harvey dived for her breast, raising it to his lips and sucking. Della cried out, one arm around his neck, holding him close.

'Yes, yes,' she moaned, so he picked up the pace, driving her higher, even as he fought off his own release. He could give her this, give her a part of himself he hadn't given anyone in twenty years. He'd let Della in emotionally. It was no wonder he felt bombarded by unfamiliar impulses.

'Della…' he groaned, his hips jerking erratically, faster and harder, his need for her boiling over.

She gasped, her fingernails digging into his shoulder as she shattered in his arms, holding him so close as her orgasm crested that all Harvey could do was crush her to his chest, bury his face against her neck and follow with a harsh cry.

'Are you okay?' he muttered, his lips against her skin, as he held her tight and came down from the high.

She nodded, retying her bikini top at the back of her neck. Slipping from her body, he helped her retie the bottoms, his insides trembling. What was she doing to him? And how would he return to his solitary life when he'd allowed her so close he feared she might be able to see through him as if he was made of glass?

Silently, they swam back under the waterfall to the main pool, holding hands as they waded ashore. Harvey glanced her way as they sat on the rocks in a shaft of tree-dappled sunlight to dry off and rehydrate. Was she, like him, moved by the intensity of what they'd just done? Was he being a fool to think she could ever take him seriously when it came to more than sex? Della was a practical, intelligent woman who knew exactly what she wanted. Could he ever be enough?

'Just to reassure you,' she said, leaning against his arm, 'because you've gone suddenly quiet—I'm on the pill. No need to worry about an unwanted consequence.' She looked up at him, the way she'd looked at him last night when he'd told her about his mother, as if he finally made sense.

'Thanks for the reassurance.' Harvey snagged her hand, raised it to his lips and pressed a kiss there. 'But I was thinking how we only have a few more days left, and how it will be extra hard to leave Fiji this time.' Because as soon as the real world encroached, they would be over. Did she still want that? Was there any part of her that wanted to see where this could lead?

She nodded, releasing a small shuddering sigh. 'I know what you mean.' She smiled at him, her expression relaxed. 'Best holiday ever.'

Harvey pulled on his T-shirt, needing to be less exposed. 'But you still want a baby, right?' he said, some inexplicable force in control of his words. 'Just not mine, obviously.' His gut twisted. With fear or some foreign ache? But he wanted Della to be happy, even if he couldn't be the man to make her so.

Della stilled, glancing over at him as if he'd asked some sort of trick question that required a considered answer. 'I do,' she said, looking down at her feet, flexing her toes in the water. 'But perhaps when I'm ready, I'll… I don't know…go it alone. Use a sperm donor. After all, I'm nearly thirty-eight. My time for finding Mr Right is running out.'

Jealous at the idea of Della with another man, Harvey pressed his lips together. Her lifestyle choices were none of his business. He certainly wasn't qualified to be the man of her dreams. It had been many years since Harvey had allowed himself to think about wanting a family. But would she truly be content to go it alone?

'That's certainly one way to go,' he said, keeping his voice light, although his throat burned. 'But isn't the adoring husband a crucial part of your dream life?'

Could he bear to watch Della walk down the aisle again now that they'd become…not friends exactly. In fact, there was no label for what they'd become. But for Harvey, it was the most meaningful connection he'd ever had. Why else would he have confided in her about his mother's abandonment? Why else was he constructing wild and improbable imaginings where he was a different man, a man worthy of Della? Especially when those imaginings put a huge part of his life—his valued place in the Wilton family—at risk.

'He was crucial...' Della rolled her eyes, looking mildly embarrassed. 'But I've kind of had my fingers burned. Maybe pushing so hard for a family was what scared off Ethan. Perhaps it's better to have part of my dream than to push for it all and end up with nothing again.'

Pricks of unease tensed Harvey's shoulders. 'Didn't he know you wanted a family before he proposed?' If Ethan had known the first thing about Della, surely it was that she'd always wanted to be a mother.

'Of course he did,' Della said, ducking her head so he could no longer see her eyes. 'But obviously he wasn't ready, or I asked for too much and ended up losing everything.'

Harvey gripped her arms, turning her to face him, his heart racing. 'Why shouldn't you have everything you want? It's not that you asked for too much, it's that Ethan sold you a lie or said one thing and then changed his mind.' His protective instincts built to a frenzy. He didn't want Della to ever doubt herself, or be scared to risk another relationship, scared to trust her judgement.

Despite being out of his depth, Harvey cupped her chin and raised her gaze back to his. 'Don't make that about you, when it was clearly his issue. You shouldn't have needed to convince him, Della. He should have understood your dreams and supported them. That's the promise he made when he married you. I was there; I heard the vows.'

Della stared, speechless, blinking up at him. Then she

dropped her gaze. 'Marriage is complex, I guess...' She shrugged, a small, vulnerable smile on her lips. 'Despite the way Brody makes it look easy.'

Harvey winced, hearing the hint of dismissal in what she left unsaid. Of course Harvey had no right to offer advice, knowing so little about commitment and nothing about marriage. She knew it. He knew it. Just because they were good together, just because he'd started to wonder if they had a future together, didn't make him some sort of instant relationship guru.

'You're right,' Harvey said, reaching for his towel to dry his legs. 'I'm the last man in the world qualified to give relationship advice. I'm not even sure I'm capable of being in one after avoiding them all these years.' He shoved his feet into his walking boots, withdrawing because he was so obviously out of his depth, and she could see right through him. She wanted a husband, a baby, and he was ill-qualified to make her the promise of even a real date.

'Maybe you're right to go it alone,' he added, stowing his towel in his backpack. 'Why wait around for some perfect guy to sweep you off your feet? If you want a baby, you should have one. Cute tiny humans. What's not to love?' Harvey shut his mouth. He had no idea what *he* wanted. But the idea of Della being a solo parent was almost as unsettling as the idea of watching her date men who were better qualified than him to be in a relationship.

Feeling powerless again, he reached for her hand and pulled her to her feet. 'Come on. Let's head back to the car. It's getting late.'

Eyeing him with curiosity, Della dressed and pulled on her backpack. They set off along the track through the forest, hand in hand once more. Harvey took some deep breaths, willing the storm inside his chest to abate. He needed to be careful. His thoughts, his imaginings were writing cheques he wasn't certain he could afford. He was the last man on Earth who should make Della any sort of promise. In a few more days, and they'd be back to their real lives. All he needed to do was silence the crazy possibilities in his head, enjoy the rest of their time together and try to ensure that their new close relationship survived once they'd each moved on.

CHAPTER ELEVEN

MONDAY MORNING, the day after their trek to Vatuwai Falls, Della awoke to find Harvey's note on her pillow.

Gone for an early run. See you at work x

She smiled, her heart fluttering with longing but her head slamming on the brakes. She headed for the shower, mulling over the intense conversation from the day before, when they'd talked about babies and her marriage and her dreams to have it all. It must have been her imagination, because Harvey had seemed…wistful? But she'd likely still been high from the way he'd touched her under the waterfall, as if he had no choice. The way he'd consumed her with his kisses and that hungry stare as he'd pushed inside her body. The way he'd confessed to always wanting her that way.

But that was just sex. Attraction. She'd felt it too, simmering away between them all these years. So why was she torturing herself with rumination when he'd also soon after warned her that he wasn't capable of being in a committed relationship? Just because she understood his heartbreaking reasons for being single didn't change the fact that he was essentially a relationship virgin, and

Della was a veteran with one failed campaign, next time searching for *the one*. And she couldn't afford to get it wrong again.

Quickly dressing, Della drank a cup of tea and dried her hair, her feelings a confused mess. But feelings, whatever shape they took, were irrelevant where Harvey was concerned. Anything beyond respect and lust was ridiculous. This was *Harvey*. Single for the past twenty years Harvey. Even if, through some major transformation, he wanted to temporarily continue their fling when they left Fiji, not only was it was physically impossible—he lived in Australia and she lived in New Zealand—it was also a huge risk to Della. If she was sleeping with Harvey, she wouldn't be dating someone else, someone who wanted to settle down, to fall in love and start a family. That was a lot to give up for *just sex*.

Trying and failing to forget about Harvey, Della arrived at the hospital. She'd barely made it to the department of surgery when an urgent call came through. She hurried to the ED, finding Harvey just ahead of her in the corridor, his hair still damp from a shower.

'What do we have?' Della asked, meeting his stare as a flurry of butterflies shifted inside her.

'Suspected stabbing, I think,' he said, shooting her a secret smile and then switching on his game face.

That's what Della needed to do. Pretend she had everything under control. Then, maybe by the time she arrived home, it would be true. Her feelings would shift into perspective and life would go back to normal, without Harvey.

Seema, the ED nurse, met them inside the resuscitation bay. 'We have a fifty-six-year-old man presenting with acute shortness of breath,' she said, handing over the ambulance report. 'Paramedics found what looks like a stab wound in his left chest wall. Erect chest X-ray results should be through any second.'

Della and Harvey rushed to opposite sides of the patient. The man was conscious, pale and sweaty and unable to talk for breathlessness. On autopilot, Della checked his vital signs on the monitor and then reached for a tourniquet. While Harvey palpated his abdomen and listened to his chest, Della drew blood from the man's arm.

'Reduced breath sounds on the left,' he told her and then added to Seema, 'I need a chest drain, please, and an urgent echo. We need to make sure the knife hasn't penetrated other structures in the chest.'

Keeping one eye on the blood pressure monitor, Della quickly labelled the blood tubes for the lab, passing them to a hospital porter. 'I've ordered a cross-match for blood transfusion,' she informed Seema. 'Have the police been called?' This obviously wasn't a self-inflicted wound.

The nurse nodded and set about replacing the empty bag of intravenous fluid feeding the drip in the patient's arm. Harvey tapped at the computer keys, bringing up the digital chest X-ray, which showed a white-out of half the left lung, indicating the presence of blood in the chest.

'Haemorthorax,' he confirmed, glancing at Della. She joined him at the monitor and took a closer look, scouring the image. 'Looks like some free air there under the diaphragm, too.' It was subtle, but free air in the abdominal cavity suggested a puncture of the stomach or intestine. 'The knife must have passed through the diaphragm.'

Harvey gave a nod, clearly on the same wavelength. Stabbing injuries to the chest, while clearly life-threatening, could also enter the peritoneal cavity and damage abdominal organs. And given the man's blood pressure was dipping dangerously low, the best way to assess trauma to the spleen, liver or kidney was an exploratory laparotomy. There was no time to hesitate.

'I'll call theatre and the anaesthetist,' Della said, reaching for the phone. 'You insert the chest drain.' The sooner they operated, the sooner they could stop any haemorrhaging and repair the perforation to the gut.

With the man booked in for an emergency laparotomy, Della quickly washed up, pulled on sterile gloves and joined Harvey on the patient's left side. Harvey swabbed the skin of the man's left chest wall and administered some local anaesthetic. Chances were there was a partial collapse of the lung along with blood inside the chest cavity. The chest drain would drain the blood and help the lung to re-expand. While Harvey carefully but expertly inserted the chest tube to drain the blood and escaped air, Della explained the man's injuries to him and consented him for theatre.

Thirty minutes later, with the patient anaesthetised and his abdomen opened up, Della found the puncture to the stomach along with a two-centimetre laceration of the liver.

'There's the hole in the diaphragm,' Harvey said, repositioning the suction to clear the operative field of blood.

'Thanks,' Della said, reaching for a suture. 'Let's sew up the liver first. Then we'll tackle the stomach.'

Harvey turned to the scrub nurse. 'Can we have a laparoscope, please?' He turned back to Della. 'We can take a look inside the chest before we close the hole in the diaphragm, make sure the pericardium is intact.'

'Good idea.' Della nodded, her eyes meeting his for a second. The echo had shown the heart and the sack around it appeared normal, but it didn't hurt to double-check while the patient was under anaesthesia.

Without getting in each other's way, they repaired the liver laceration and stitched up the stomach perforation. Operating together had become so intuitive now, Della worried that she might forget how to do it alone when their time in Fiji was over. But she couldn't rely on Harvey for anything. Reality was calling. By the end of this week, he'd go his way and she'd go hers, and this, *them*, would be over.

She waited for the rush of relief, but it didn't come. Perhaps that was simply because they still had one more test to get through before they were truly out of the woods when it came to moving on: Jack's naming day. She would see Harvey again in a couple of weeks. It was hard to believe that she wouldn't want him still. But indulging would only delay the inevitable, and she'd be foolish to endlessly pursue a dead end. She couldn't have Harvey forever, so it was best to make a clean break after Fiji. To try and switch off the constant need for him. To fill her thoughts with something other than Harvey and how he made her feel as if she'd been alone for long enough, that as long as she kept her eye on the prize, she *could* achieve her dreams.

An hour later, with the surgery complete and the patient headed to the surgical ward, they de-gowned, washed up and headed for the staff room.

'I need tea,' Della said, flicking on the kettle. Maybe it was a good idea to start weaning herself off Harvey now, before she became any more attached.

Harvey passed Della the tea bags, his stare distracted. 'Let's sit down for a few minutes. I have something to tell you.' He busied himself with making black coffee, his expression serious so Della's nerves fluttered in her chest.

'Oh, oh. That sounds…ominous.' Della added milk to her tea, her mind unhelpfully filling in the blanks. Was he flying home early as she'd teased that day they'd agreed to their fling? Given that she'd literally just decided to start a controlled exit, that shouldn't matter, but her stomach took a sickening dive nonetheless, telling her she was already in trouble.

'I think it's good news,' Harvey said, leading the way to two comfy armchairs in the corner of the staff room.

'What is it?' Della asked impatiently, taking a seat.

'I checked my work emails this morning.' Harvey settled into the chair next to her and placed his coffee on a side table. 'Dr Jones, one of my senior colleagues, has announced his retirement.' His stare met hers, so she saw a flicker of excitement there. 'They'll be appointing his replacement, if you're interested.'

His tone was casual, but Della stilled, her heart racing with both a surge of excitement and a greater sense of panic. Before Fiji, before she'd slept with Harvey again, before she'd seen the other side of him, a job back in her native Melbourne doing what she loved would have been a dream come true. But now…the idea of working in Harvey's department came with extra considerations. Could she see him every day and get over him, over this fling, at the same time?

'You don't like the idea,' he said, his voice flat.

'It's not that.' Della touched his arm. 'I'm thinking,'

she hedged, her mind racing as fast as her pulse. 'Has the job even been advertised yet?'

'Not yet,' Harvey confirmed, ignoring his coffee while he observed her intently. 'But there have to be some perks when you're sleeping with the head of the department.' He flashed her a cheeky wink. 'I'm giving you advanced warning, before the job goes public.'

'There's no guarantee I'd get it, of course,' she mumbled, unable to meet his stare. Maybe the fact that a big part of her loved the idea was reason in itself to be cautious. Yes, their time in Fiji had proved that when it came to their jobs, they could get along just fine. But that was with a set expiration date for the end of their fling. It would be a very different story if their physical relationship limped along back in Melbourne, until one of them—Della because she wanted more, or Harvey because he didn't—broke it off. And what then?

Could she continue to take the only part of him on offer, sex, knowing he was too scared to ever consider having a real relationship? Could she work in the same department as Harvey every day and watch him return to his single life? Could she see him socially with her family and still manage to keep her own feelings at bay? Because she could not fall for Harvey Ward. They wanted different things. She'd be humiliated again. Hurt. And she'd only have herself to blame for making the same mistake twice.

'Hmm…' she offered, 'perhaps I'm just too tired to think straight. We have been living on very little sleep for a week.' Della tried to smile, but it felt like a grimace. 'Perhaps we should sleep alone tonight and catch up.' She felt sick. Suddenly she had no idea what she wanted, but some distance, some time away from Harvey to think, might help.

'Of course…' he said, concern and guilt hovering in his stare. Then he frowned, glanced down at his hands. 'I'll be honest. I thought you'd be a little more enthusiastic about the job. After the hard time you gave me three years ago, I assumed moving back to Melbourne was still something you really wanted.'

'It *is* something I want,' Della said unconvincingly. 'I'm just considering all the implications.'

'What implications?' His frown deepened.

'You know…' Della squirmed. 'Us, working together.' There was a lot to think about. It wasn't a decision she could rush, not if she hoped to protect herself in the process.

'We've managed to do that successfully for over a week, Della.' Harvey shrugged, a flicker of hurt in his eyes. 'Why would Melbourne be any different?'

Della swallowed. That was exactly her point—it *wouldn't* be any different. With the exception of their fling being over, everything would be the same. Harvey would still be avoiding relationships, because on some level he was scared to be vulnerable after being abandoned by his mother and losing Alice. And Della wanted a relationship, but would still be terrified to pin all her dreams on another person in case she got it wrong again. But the fact that Harvey was suggesting them working together would be easy told Della exactly where his head was. For him, it was straightforward. The fling would be over, business as usual, no problem. Whereas Della already suspected she'd take longer to adjust, that her feelings, her desire for him, would take time to switch off.

Hoping the wild flutter of her pulse wasn't obvious, Della breathed through her fear and met his stare. 'It's not that we *couldn't* successfully work together, Harvey. It's just… It would be intense after…you know…everything we've shared here. It will take some time to adjust to going back to what we were before. That's all.'

She couldn't bring herself to call them friends. She had a sneaking suspicion that Harvey would always be tempting. She'd known going into this fling that it was temporary, but now that it was almost over, now that she understood him, now that she saw he might be too broken to allow himself to be happy, to believe he was loveable, there was a part of Della that couldn't help but wonder *what if*?

What if he could see that he was worthy of being loved? What if he overcame his fear and gave a real relationship a shot? What if she and Harvey *could* work?

'I think we could make it work,' he said, as if reading her mind. But where she was talking about a relationship between them, he meant them working together in the same department.

Della almost laughed at how out of sync they were, but instead nodded vaguely, her fatigue weighing heavily. Of course she was so much more invested emotionally than Harvey. He'd spent twenty years holding people away, whereas she wore her *heart on her sleeve*, as he'd said. Just because he'd told her about Alice and his mother didn't make Della special. He was still putting up emotional barriers, and if she wasn't very careful, she'd make a fool of herself and get hurt.

'I'd hate our fling to be the reason you didn't apply,'

he pushed, making it sound so easy, so cold and clinical. 'I know how much you miss being close to your family.'

Della nodded, her heart sinking. That was Harvey— his mind on the fling, confident that when it was over, he'd just slip back into his single life. But he'd warned her that he was no good at relationships. He'd abandoned messy emotions years ago, because they made him feel powerless. If she'd ignored the obvious signposts, that was *her* problem.

'Well, I'll definitely look out for the job ad,' she said. 'Thanks for the heads-up.'

'Great,' he said, sounding less certain than before.

Della swallowed the lump in her throat, glugged her tea and pasted on a bright smile she was far from feeling. He seemed merely worried about a bit of workplace awkwardness, given the amount of sex they'd had. He hadn't mentioned them continuing to see each other after Fiji, but then, what did she expect? And was she really going to miss out on her dream job again because of Harvey, when all she needed to do was put this fling behind her as easily?

'I might head back to the emergency department,' Della said, standing. 'See what's happening before I call it a day. You finish your coffee.'

He nodded, clearly bewildered, and she fled, needing some distance. As she walked, she gave herself a stern talking to. Clearly Harvey saw no problems with them working together, because he fully intended to return to his old life. It was only soppy, romantic Della who was overthinking it with improbable what-ifs.

Even if by some miracle, Harvey wanted a real relationship, when it came to commitment, he was beyond rusty. Della couldn't afford to carry him while he tried a relationship on for size. Nor, with time to build her dreams running out, could she afford to be wrong again about anyone, including Harvey.

Harvey walked into the ED, guilt and confusion still knotting his insides. Della *had* looked tired. Was his constant need for her selfish? Their time together in Fiji had been intense. Perhaps she was right. Perhaps a night in their own beds would help them both achieve some clarity.

So why did he feel so crushed, as if Della was already withdrawing from him, despite the fact they still had three nights of their holiday left? He glanced around, hoping to spy her, as if one of her smiles would settle the doubts coiling inside him. Her tepid reaction to his news of a job vacancy had completely swept his feet from under him. He'd assumed she'd be overjoyed to come home, not hesitant. But maybe she was right to apply the brakes. Maybe he should proceed with caution, too. After all, a job in his department represented a significant move for Della, and seeing her every day at work would be an adjustment for them both. Maybe Harvey was too invested in the idea of them working together long-term, whereas Della intended for them to return to the way they were. Maybe he was jumping the gun when he should be preparing himself for the end of their fling instead.

A growing sense of foreboding urged him onwards in his search. If he only knew what she was thinking... He found Della in resus with a patient, a boy around ten years old, and his father. His heart lurched at the sight of her as if they'd been estranged for years, not minutes.

As he approached, Della looked up with no evidence

of her earlier doubts. 'Dr Ward, this is Taito. He fell from his trampoline this afternoon. I was just explaining to Dad that he has a fractured femur.'

The boy moaned in pain. Harvey greeted the patient and his father, stepping close to Della to examine the X-ray on the screen, while a trickle of relief calmed his pulse.

'Mid-shaft, spiral fracture,' she said to Harvey, placing a butterfly needle in the crook of Taito's left arm before addressing the boy. 'I'm going to give you some more medicine for the pain.' She injected the painkillers slowly into the vein and then touched the boy's shoulder in comfort, her expression full of her signature compassion.

Harvey's pulse bounded as he watched her work. Della was such a caring person, that big heart of hers making her so hard to resist. No wonder he was struggling.

A fresh wave of panic struck him. He wanted more time.

'Skin traction will help with pain relief,' Harvey said, staring into her eyes, searching for her true feelings, desperate to know how she felt about him to help him understand what was going on inside his own head.

'I'll get that organised with Seema,' she said, holding his eye contact as if silently communicating something he was too confused to see.

'Want me to ring the on-call orthopaedic reg?' he asked, needing to be near her because she made him feel better, but also aware that she was nearing the end of a long day, and he could help out.

'Yes, please,' she said, flicking him a look of gratitude. 'I'll meet you in the office shortly.'

Harvey used the phone in the doctors' office to speak

to his orthopaedic colleague, making the referral. Taito's fracture would need internal fixation surgery, but he and Della could pass the case on. He'd not long hung up the phone when Della appeared.

'Long day…' she said, taking the seat beside his to add a note to the patient's file.

'How is Taito?' he asked, wishing he could massage her shoulders, run her bath and pour her a glass of wine. But they'd agreed to spend the night apart.

'He fell asleep as soon as the painkillers kicked in. His poor father felt so guilty.' She turned to face him, her stare full of uncertainty, or perhaps he was just imagining it.

Harvey reached for her hand and wrapped his fingers around hers. 'Why don't you go home, have a relax in the bath, a glass of wine and an early night.'

'Sounds heavenly,' Della said, her stare searching his so he witnessed her doubts. She sighed. Then, without warning, she leaned close and pressed her lips to his, her body sagging against his chest.

'What was that for?' Harvey asked when she pulled back, his hand cupping her face.

'No reason,' she said with a small frown, 'other than I wanted to kiss you. In a few days' time I won't be able to.'

Harvey's pulse thudded harder, the reminder that their time in Fiji would soon be over releasing another cascade of panic. Della leaned in again, slid her fingers through his hair and kissed him slowly and thoroughly as if she was memorising the feel of his lips against hers for when this was over. Harvey gripped her upper arms and kissed her back, more confused than ever but determined to take every scrap of her she would allow in the time they had left.

When they parted, each breathing hard, she blinked up at him. 'Come home with me,' she whispered. Her eyes were heavy, her pupils dilating.

Excitement energised Harvey's body, mocking his attempts to stay in control of his thoughts and how she made him feel. 'I thought you were tired.' He brushed the hair back from her face.

Suddenly he didn't care about preparing himself for the end of their fling. He wanted as much of Della as he could get until they left the island. Maybe by then, he'd have his conflicted feelings all figured out.

'I am, but I don't care.' She took his hand and dropped her gaze. 'It's just struck me that we only have a few nights left, and I don't want to waste a single second.' She met his stare, hers bold. 'I don't want to have regrets when I leave here.'

Harvey tilted up her chin and brushed her lips with his. 'Neither do I.' He would immerse himself in this relationship until the last minute. Surely by then, a way forward would present itself.

'Let's go,' he said, logging off from the computer. 'I'll run you that bath and pour you a glass of wine.'

'Harvey,' she said, reaching for his arm so he stilled. 'Thanks for thinking of me for the job. I will seriously consider it.'

He nodded, wanting to crush her in his arms and beg her to apply, but maybe Della could see pitfalls he hadn't even considered. 'You're welcome, Della.' Considering her for a colleague was no hardship, given he thought about her every minute of every day. And despite all the reasons for caution, he couldn't see that abating anytime soon.

CHAPTER TWELVE

Two days later, jittery with nerves, Harvey walked behind Della, his hands covering her eyes as he guided her
into the luxury villa he'd booked for their final night in
Fiji.

'Ready?' he asked, sucking in the scent of her freshly
washed hair and her light floral perfume, his heart thump-
ing with bittersweet excitement.

Della nodded, her hand gripping his arm. 'You'd better not have brought me to see one of those giant coconut
crabs, because that's not funny.'

'Would I do that to you? You hate crabs,' Harvey said,
his doubts building because romance wasn't his strong
point. 'Now, keep your eyes closed until I say so.' He
removed his hands from her eyes and stepped around
Della, positioning himself so he could see her reaction.
'Okay, open them.'

Della blinked, quickly glanced his way and then took
in the room, which was scattered with flickering tea light
candles. The French doors opened to reveal their own private veranda with an in-ground infinity-edged spa pool
that overlooked the sea views.

Her eyes widened, and her hands covered her mouth.
'Oh... It's so beautiful. This is so thoughtful of you,

Harvey.' She reached for him, her smile worth a hundred words.

Harvey snaked his arm around her waist, drawing her into his arms, relief flooding his system. 'We've had such a busy week, we deserve a treat on our last night. Do you want to have a soak in the spa before we eat?'

'Definitely,' she said, her eyes full of excitement and laughter as she kicked off her sandals and reached for the hem of her dress. Underneath, she wore the pink bikini he loved. While Della climbed in the spa, Harvey hastily tossed aside his shirt, poured two glasses of wine and then joined her.

The water was warm, the sounds of the sea and the Fijian insect life from the surrounding forest soothing background noise. But not even Della's obvious delight could chase off the hollowness deep at the centre of his chest. A huge part of him didn't want to go home. So many times this week, he'd almost raised the subject of them seeing where this relationship could go, and each time, he'd chickened out, kept his mouth shut, his doubts that he could form a committed relationship building. But his head couldn't seem to let the idea go.

'To two weeks in paradise,' Harvey said, making a toast to remind her how far they'd come in such a short time.

Della touched her glass to his, her eyes bright. 'Who'd have thought that being stuck with each other would turn out to be so…rejuvenating.' Before he could comment, she playfully sat astride his lap, resting her arms on his shoulders, leaning in to press a kiss to his lips.

Harvey savoured the contact, his heart thudding wildly. Della seemed to be handling their final night better than him, not that it was a competition. But where he was desperate to talk about the future, to voice his feelings and find out what she was thinking, Della seemed to be intent on keeping things light. It left him wondering if his instincts were way off. That if he tried to talk to her about them, she might dismiss him out of hand.

He swallowed hard as she pulled back, trying not to get lost in her stare. 'So, how do you want to play it?' he asked, his voice strangled with lust and confusion. Before he got too carried away by her touch, her kisses, that seductive look in her eyes, he at least wanted to address Jack's naming day in a fortnight, when they would definitely see each other again.

'Play what?' She shifted on his lap, the position putting her breasts in his line of vision, which was very distracting.

'Us,' he choked out, 'at Jack's naming day, with your family.'

Della tangled her fingers in his hair and tilted his head back, sliding her lips from his earlobe to his jaw, her touch speeding up his already erratic pulse. 'Well, given we agreed to leave *us* behind when we left Fiji, we'll find a way.'

His heart sank further. He closed his eyes, arousal a fire in his blood as she trailed her lips down the side of his neck. But his words, his yearning wanted an outlet before it was too late and they'd succumbed to this endless need for each other. 'But don't you think one of your family—probably Brody, let's be honest—will be able to tell something is different with us?'

It would be a miracle if Harvey managed to keep his eyes off Della when they next met, and if he looked at her, surely someone would be able to see what he was too scared to articulate—how he had feelings for Della he had no idea what to do with. But the two of them exploring more than sex felt ludicrous. An outrageous and risky fantasy. He'd been single by choice for twenty years, and Della... Della was a hearts and flowers romantic who deserved to have her every wish come true. How could a man like him ever be good enough?

What did Harvey know about long-term commitment? What would he have to offer this incredible woman? Even if she did want him, could he step up and be what she needed, or would he ruin everything if he tried, losing people he considered family?

'That's easy.' Della sat back, her expression transparent as she placed her wineglass on the edge of the spa. 'We'll throw Brody off the scent. I'll make a few digs at you, and you can goad me into an argument, perhaps over the wine. No one will ever know.' She chuckled, pressed her lips back to his, and writhed on his lap so he struggled to think of anything beyond how much he wanted her. But beneath the arousal, his stomach knotted.

He didn't want Della and him to revert to the strangers of old, bickering as if these two unexpected and passionate weeks hadn't happened. But Della was obviously happy to leave this, them, behind. Whereas Harvey...? He wasn't sure which way was up, but he was terrified that he'd never be able to switch off this physical craving. He'd found something with her here in Fiji. Nothing as mundane as friendship, more like an intense connection someplace way beyond friends. Mutual acceptance and respect and...obsession. There was no point trying to pretend. He thought about her all the time, wanted to be around her every moment of every day. For the first time in years, he'd developed deep feelings for a woman, a woman who didn't, *couldn't*, feel the same way about him. A woman he needed to protect from the kind of man he'd become, because she deserved so much more than he could give.

The familiar taste of rejection and failure burned his throat, so he held her closer, tighter. 'Do you think we can pull it off?' he asked, placing his wineglass beside hers. 'Not the bickering for Brody's sake, but...you know...the clean break?' His heart raced as if he was a teenager with a crush, asking for a girl's number. He held his breath balanced on the edge of a knife. Harvey had never been less certain of anything in his life or more out of control. But Della did this to him, left him powerless until he wasn't sure whether to run from the feeling or push through it to the brave new world on the other side.

Della stilled, staring down at him with a frown. 'I think we'll be okay. After all, we live in different countries.' She smiled, her fingers moving restlessly through his hair.

Was she making light of their split to protect herself or to let Harvey off the hook? Because they both knew he was in foreign waters here, wanting more than sex. He had no idea what more would even look like for them. He didn't want this fling to end, but nor was he certain he could make her the kind of promises he knew she wanted and deserved after so many years of shutting down his feelings. Was he simply being selfish by trying to hold on? Would he be the ultimate loser if he tried and failed?

'As easy as that, huh?' he asked, barely able to breathe, he was so confused and conflicted. And he hadn't missed the fact that she'd yet to confirm if she was applying for the job in Melbourne.

She frowned, her stare shifting between his eyes. 'It'll be an adjustment. I'll miss this.' Shifting her hips on his lap, she brushed his lips with hers.

Harvey's hands glided from her back to her hips, holding her still. Every move she made, her curves and softness filling his arms were torture to his strung-out body. He wanted to crush her to his chest and pleasure her over and over again until dawn when they needed to leave for the airport. Maybe then, he'd have worked her fully out of his system and everything would make sense. Maybe then, Della would look at him the way she had under the waterfall, as if he, broken, unworthy Harvey, might just be the answer to her dreams. But who was he trying to kid?

'I'll miss this too, Della,' he said, his throat raw with longing. *I'll miss you.* Gripping her waist, he buried his face against her breasts, over the beat of her heart. Now that their last night together was here, he wanted to rewind time. To go back to the start of their two weeks. Or better still, to go back twenty years and be a different man, one who'd overcome his grief and the ingrained belief that there was something unlovable about him and who deserved Della. One who understood that losing Alice, losing his mother's love, had nothing to do with him and everything to do with the unfair randomness of life and the selfish choices of others.

Della was right. He wasn't that powerless kid anymore. Except she made him feel that way, as if one wrong move would shatter the safe, predicable existence he'd clung to most of his adult life. He'd wasted so much time fighting his desire for this woman, when now it was all he could think about.

Della stroked his hair, and he held her tighter. He didn't want their last night to be only about desire. He needed to know Fiji had meant something to her, because it meant something to him.

'Would you have dated me when we first met?' he asked, looking up. 'If I'd been ready to ask you and you'd been single? If I hadn't been grieving and you weren't my best friend's sister?' Regret was pointless. Time travel impossible. But he needed to know that he hadn't been alone in imagining the shadow of what might have been between them all this time.

Della froze, her stare flitting. 'I… I don't know. Perhaps I would… It wasn't that I didn't fancy you, just that we've always wanted different things.'

Harvey nodded, too confused to explain that he wasn't sure what he wanted anymore. Somehow, it was easier to admit how he'd felt about her when they'd first met than how he felt now, tonight. But instinct told him Della was preparing to walk away, and he couldn't blame her. What did he have to offer? Just himself, as lacking as he was?

'I know the timing was wrong for us both, but part of me wishes I'd asked you back then,' he said, his voice thick with emotion. 'Who knows how life might have turned out differently if I had?'

Confused, her frown deepened, her fingers stilling in his hair. 'It's in the past. We can't change it.'

'Right. I guess I wanted you to know that I've always fancied you. I just wasn't ready for a relationship. And even twenty years ago, despite being a bit of a jerk, I was smart enough to know that hurting you would have cost me nearly everything I had—you, Brody, your mum and dad.'

'Harvey…' she whispered, resting her forehead against his, but somehow still seeing right through him. 'You know it wasn't your fault, don't you?'

Harvey froze, his pulse flying. Why hadn't he just seduced her instead of trying to verbalise the storm raging inside him?

'Not your parents' divorce,' she continued, 'or your mother choosing to leave, or Alice's accident.'

'I know.' Those events weren't his fault, but they had shaped him, made him someone who valued emotional control over all else. And look where that had led.

'And you have nothing to prove anymore,' she said, brushing his lips with hers. 'You're in control of your own life.'

The change of subject felt like a goodbye, a pep talk, a final note to see him on his way. Crushed by her emotional withdrawal, Harvey held her tight, pressing his face against her chest. He didn't want her to fix him. He wanted her to want him. To choose him over all men. But he'd seen the same look in her eyes when he'd encouraged her to apply for the Melbourne job. If he pushed for more than this fling, he might discover that he could never be what Della needed, that she wanted so much more than he was capable of. Could he live with that knowledge when he had to live with her in his life?

'Let's go to bed,' she whispered, tilting his head back, her lips finding his, parting, caressing, while her hips rocked on his lap.

Clinging to the distraction of her touch, he gazed up at her. Maybe she was right to remind him this was about pleasure. Maybe this was the only part of her he could have. Maybe once he was away from her, he'd move on as easily as she predicted. Harvey steeled himself against the pleasure her kisses always delivered, his hands cupping her breasts to coax out those moans he loved.

Della gasped, her eyes glazed with arousal as he thumbed her nipples erect. Because he was raw and exposed and ravenous for her, as always, he chased her lips with his. Their tongues met and duelled as their kisses deepened out of control. He might not be able to give her a ring, a family, that white picket fence dream, but he could give her this. Make tonight one she'd always remember.

Harvey slipped his hand between her legs, inside her bikini bottoms, and stroked her. Della broke free of their kiss to stare down at him, her pupils dilating with arousal. Emotions fluttered through her eyes. Arousal, uncertainty, perhaps even fear. But of course she would be scared to expect anything from him, scared to trust that he could be more than a good time, and she was right. The powerless feeling he detested returned. He couldn't let her down. He couldn't lose Della or the other Wiltons from his life. Better to let her go now and keep a part of her forever than to risk losing everything.

Harvey stroked her faster, one arm holding her around her waist. She rode his hand, her eyes on his and her arms braced on his shoulders.

'Kiss me,' he said, because he wanted to forget that this would be the last time he touched her, the last time he held her in his bed and awoke to the scent of her perfume on his pillow.

She whimpered, grasped his neck and lowered her

mouth to his. Her hips bucked. He stroked her faster, slid his fingers inside her and braced himself against her wild kisses.

'If you had asked me twenty years ago,' she panted after pulling away, 'I would have said yes.'

Triumph soared in Harvey's chest. He tugged down her bikini top and bent his head, captured her exposed nipple, sucking. She cried out her climax, her slippery body bucking against his under the water. Harvey held her close. Her heart thudded against his cheek where he'd crushed her in his arms. She whimpered and he slid his hand from between her legs, wrapping both arms around her, certain that he should never let her go in case it became the biggest mistake of his life.

Hours later, Della clung to Harvey as the dying cries of her orgasm echoed around the room. The moonlight shone through the window of their bure, streaking the sumptuous bed with surreal shafts of light. She kissed him, snatching breaths between surges of her tongue against his. The entire night, from the moment he'd excitedly collected her and her cases from the staff bungalow at the hospital to when he'd made love to her over and over again, carried a fantastical dreamlike quality. And Della was scared to wake up.

Harvey groaned, tore his mouth from hers and collapsed on top of her, his body racked with the spasms of his climax as he crushed her close, so close she almost lost her breath.

'We have to stop,' Della said, panting, pushing his sweaty hair back from his face. 'We have to stop before we kill each other like those horny mice.' Her plea was feeble, born of exhaustion more than a desire to stop. The night had been both endless and too short. Every time one of them dozed off, the other would reach for them again, their touch, their kisses quickly escalating as if they were both intent on outrunning the passage of time. But it was as if they'd missed their chance twenty years ago, and they both knew it.

Harvey slid from her body and rolled to the side, drawing her onto his chest. He pressed his lips to her head, his arms banded around her shoulders. 'I don't want to stop. I can't seem to.'

Della nodded, her eyelids heavy. 'Me neither.' But as the pleasure subsided, the heavy ache in her chest returned. Her flight to Auckland was leaving in four hours. She could sleep on the plane. If she closed her eyes now, if she fell asleep, their relationship would be over when she awoke, and a part of her never wanted that moment to come.

Harvey's words from earlier scratched at the closed door in her mind. They'd sounded like regrets. But surely Harvey hadn't changed his mind about staying single? He couldn't possibly want a relationship. He didn't do those. Perhaps Della was simply seeing what she wanted to see.

Scared that she was projecting her own feelings onto him, Della closed her eyes. She'd spent all week preparing for this night, their last, holding something back, refusing to rely on her intuition, focussed on the end goal: leaving Fiji and moving on from their fling. Because Harvey might have regrets—everyone did to some extent—but he still wasn't ready to change. Maybe he was too broken to allow himself to be loved. Maybe, because of his mother, he felt inherently unworthy of love. But Della needed to be strong. This time, she couldn't afford to be wrong or settle for a relationship with misaligned expectations. This time, she had to get it right.

'Can I call you from Australia?' he asked, his voice husky with lack of sleep. 'I won't just miss the sex. I'll miss you, too.'

Della's heart fluttered painfully at his words. It had been an intense fortnight. Adjusting to their new reality would feel strange for a while. But could she be Harvey's friend, knowing how close she'd come to falling for him? If they talked, their emotional connection would deepen, at least for Della. Could she then keep her feelings at bay the way she'd tried to every night in his arms this week, or would missing him, craving him, cause those feelings to overwhelm her? Wasn't a clean break the only sure-fire way to protect her heart? After all, she'd tried and failed miserably to wean herself off sleeping with Harvey.

'I don't know, Harvey.' She felt him tense, and her arms reflexively tightened around his chest. 'I'll be honest, I'll struggle to be your friend at the moment.' She felt the thud of his heart under her cheek and went on. 'There's just so much water under the bridge when it comes to us. If we talk, I may weaken next time I see you and end up seducing you again. You know how weak my willpower is.' The dash of humour was intended to soften the blow, but Della had never felt less like smiling, because every word was true and laced with fear.

'Would that be so terrible?' He pressed his lips to the top of her head. 'When we're not bickering, we're very good together.'

Della blinked, her eyes stinging. 'Of course it wouldn't

be terrible. But this time here with you has made me realise that maybe I am ready to start dating again. That husband I'm after isn't going to just land in my lap, so I probably need to get out there and find him.'

All Harvey was offering was another night in his bed. As tempting as that was, she'd want so much more. She'd want another night and another and another. Then she'd fall in love with him and want him to be the man of her dreams. Would he ever be ready for that? And could Della afford to put those dreams on hold again and wait around on the off chance that he might change his mind?

He'd told her to be uncompromising when it came to her next relationship, and he was right. If they tried to drag this physical fling out, she'd be forced to one day make the tough choice: amazing sex with Harvey or having it all with someone else. She'd hate herself if she reached her expiration date like all his other women. Because it would be so easy to allow herself to fall in love with the Harvey she'd come to know in Fiji. Maybe they were better off as friends, after all.

'I've had a wonderful time. I'll never forget it.' Gripping his face, she pressed her lips to his, ignoring the flicker of disappointment in his dark stare. She felt it too. It was hard to give up something so good. But Della needed to be selfish, to trust her gut and go after what she wanted, to have it all.

'Me neither,' he said hesitantly.

'And if I get the job in your department, we might end up working together again.' Maybe friends and colleagues were for the best. So why did it suddenly feel like a second-rate consolation prize?

He offered her a smile tinged with sadness she didn't want to acknowledge. 'I'd like that. I really hope you'll apply.'

Della nodded, the burn in her chest, the plummeting of her stomach leaving her to wonder just how she would work with Harvey every day and not want him. Tonight had almost broken her. Their out-of-control need for each other was so profound, she wondered how she would survive the sexual drought to come.

But survive it she must.

CHAPTER THIRTEEN

Two weeks later.

HARVEY SMOOTHED A nervous hand down the front of his polo shirt and yanked open his front door, his heart lurching at the wonderful sight of Della on his doorstep. His pulse galloped so fast he worried he might pass out.

'Della. You look…nice.' *Nice?* Two weeks away from her, pining and picking up the phone to call her, and stalking her social media accounts to see if she was dating anyone, and *nice* was the best he could do?

Before he could reach for her and kiss her, she stepped over the threshold, holding out a bottle of red wine like a shield. 'I brought you a lovely New Zealand Pinot Noir. If you don't like it, you can serve it to Brody. He'll drink anything,' she said, breezing past him without so much as a proper glance.

She headed for the kitchen, where her family were already gathered, leaving Harvey stunned and confused. He closed the door, his stomach in his shoes and his legs threatening to collapse. That wasn't the reunion he'd expected, the reunion he'd played out in his mind on a daily basis. The one where he kissed her, told her that *friends* wasn't working for him, that missing her had made him realise for the first time in twenty years he wanted a real relationship, with *her*, and then kissed her once more. All it had taken to bring about this massive realisation was a bit of physical distance. Without her body asleep next to his, the bed felt too big. Without her smile, her laughter, the challenge in her eyes, beautiful Melbourne seemed drab. Without Della to bounce ideas off, even his work seemed...mundane.

But clearly Della was still set on the charade for her family, acting as if Fiji hadn't happened. And Harvey could understand. He didn't want to answer any questions about them until he'd had a chance to talk to Della alone.

Cursing the wisdom of hosting a barbecue for the Wiltons the night Della had arrived from Auckland, Harvey joined them in his kitchen. He should have met her at the airport, taken her out to dinner instead, kissed her until her eyes glazed with passion and made love to her all night long just to prove that they could never be just friends. That colleagues alone wouldn't work either, because he wanted her more, not less, than when they'd been in Fiji. But what did Della want, and what if it wasn't him?

Thinking back to their reserved farewell kiss in Nadi Airport, just before he'd boarded one plane to Melbourne and Della another to Auckland, Harvey glanced her way. He understood that she'd been protecting herself on that final night when he'd tried to push for more. He was a big risk for someone who wanted lifelong commitment. But was that enough reason for them to completely give up on something so good? If she'd only give him a chance, he'd show her that his feelings were genuine. That he was ready to let her in and try to be what she needed.

Brody kissed his sister on the cheek, refusing to take

the bottle of wine Harvey set in front of him. 'Not for me. I'm a changed man.' He cast a nervous glance at his wife, who was conspicuously sipping a soft drink. 'Now that Dells is here,' Brody continued, 'we may as well tell you all—Amy is pregnant again. Jack's having a little sister!'

Jenny Wilton hugged her daughter-in-law, and Brody's dad, Graham, shifted Jack in his arms to embrace his son. Congratulations flew. But while Harvey was happy for his friend, his eyes were glued to Della's reaction.

She stood frozen, her eyes blinking rapidly as if she was fighting tears. Harvey's heart jolted in his chest. He'd never seen Della cry. His arms ached to hold her, to whisper how much he'd missed her these endless two weeks, to kiss her and make her a hundred promises that might put a smile back on her face. But what if his promises weren't enough? What if she stonewalled him again like she had in Fiji?

'I'm so happy for you,' she said bravely, snapping out of her trance to hug Amy and then Brody.

'It's early days,' Amy said, laughing, 'and we don't know if it's a sister or brother yet, but Brody seems to think he's telepathic.'

To give himself something to do beyond clearing the house of the other Wiltons so he could be alone with Della, Harvey collected a bottle of fizz from the fridge and popped the cork. 'Just a drop to celebrate,' he said, handing a grinning Brody a glass.

Harvey offered Della a glass of champagne, trying to catch her eye, but she was avoiding looking at him. Instead she declined, putting her arm around Amy's waist. 'I'll abstain in solidarity with Amy, seeing as Brody has no willpower.'

The excited chatter continued as the Wiltons drifted outside to the deck. Why wouldn't she look at him? Yes, they'd agreed to a clean break—he'd done what she asked and not called—agreed to act normal in front of Della's family. The last thing they needed were intrusive questions when their relationship was so...fragile. But how could she act as if that fortnight in Fiji had never happened, when a huge part of Harvey wanted to announce to the world that he wanted her in his life? Not as a friend or a colleague, but as a partner.

Harvey's stomach twisted with doubt. Maybe Della wasn't as sure about him as he was about her. Maybe she wanted more than she believed he could offer. Maybe if he pushed her again, he might ruin what they already had and lose her from his life. That wasn't an option.

'So, what did Harvey get up to in Fiji, sis?' Brody asked, flicking Harvey a knowing look. 'Any wild nights to report? Did he leave a trail of broken hearts scattered all over the islands?'

'Don't ask me,' Della snapped, avoiding Harvey's stare. 'Ask him. He's *your* friend.'

It was the kind of thing she might have said before Fiji, before they'd become lovers, before he'd opened up to her about his mother in a way he'd never done with anyone else. It was part of the act they'd agreed to, so why did Harvey feel as if she'd physically punched him in the gut?

'Oh, I have asked him,' Brody said playfully, completely missing the tension between Harvey and Della, 'but he's been uncharacteristically tight-lipped. There must have been someone, though. He hasn't had so much as a coffee date since he's been back. If I didn't know better, I'd say he'd met someone he actually cared about.'

Harvey's entire body tensed as he willed Della to look his way. He *had* met someone he cared about—*her*. He wanted her to want him, to fight for him, not disown him. He wanted to matter to her enough that she chose him, here and now in front of her family, people he also considered *his* family. But what if her apparent coldness wasn't an act? What if she'd easily reverted to her feelings of contempt now that their fling was done? What if everything he'd confided in her, everything they'd shared, meant nothing?

Feeling nauseous, Harvey shot Brody a warning a look. Normally he wouldn't care about being the butt of his friend's joke. But something seemed off with Della. Perhaps she was upset about her brother's announcement.

'Oh, I doubt it,' Della said, finally glancing Harvey's way. 'You know what they say—a leopard never changes its spots.' Her expression was another physical blow—confusion, anguish, a flicker of longing gone before Harvey could be certain of it. She turned back to Brody. 'But I was there to work, not to catalogue your friend's female cast-offs.' Spinning on her heel, she joined her parents, who were sitting with Jack on the grass. On seeing his aunt, Jack held out his chubby fists. Della swung him up into her arms, her face beaming with the first genuine smile of the evening.

Harvey's entire body sagged, his pulse thrumming with hunger. He wanted Della to look at *him* that way. He didn't want to play it cool. He didn't care about awkward questions. He'd rather announce to her family that he wanted her to move back to Melbourne so they could try and have a proper relationship.

Hearing how absurd and inadequate his solution

sounded in his head, Harvey deflated. How could Della and he, of all men, work out when she was already way ahead of him, looking for love, a husband, a family of her own? She'd rejected his attempts to start a conversation about them back in Fiji, as good as telling him he wasn't relationship material. He wasn't good enough for her. Felling utterly powerless, he glanced at Brody and winced.

'What on Earth did you do this time to upset Della?' Brody asked sheepishly, as if at last he was finally picking up on the tension between them, the weird dynamic that didn't quite ring true.

Harvey shrugged, his chest hollow, all the excitement of seeing Della again draining away. 'Just existed, I think, mate. Same as usual.'

Only there was one additional thing that wasn't usual—the way he felt inside, as if he'd explode unless he could convince Della to hear him out. With a sickening lurch of his stomach, Harvey realised he might already be falling in love with Della, and it wasn't going to be anywhere near enough.

Della stacked the final plate into the dishwasher, her head all over the place and heart aching. Outside, happy conversations and laughter of her family swirled around. Tomorrow, Jack's naming day would be a joyous occasion, but her smiles felt insincere, and she could barely look at Harvey, so strong was the desire to hurl herself into his arms and make him want her forever.

Della swallowed down the sense of panic. The past two weeks without him had been a living hell. She'd been wrong; the physical distance, the lack of contact, the clean break…*nothing* had helped her get over their fling. *Nothing* was back to normal. Her feelings, the ones she'd tried to deny and sweep under the rug in Fiji, were bigger than ever, especially now that she'd seen Harvey again. The hurt in his eyes when she'd tried to throw Brody off the scent had crushed her.

With a trembling hand, she closed the dishwasher and went in search of Harvey's bathroom. She needed a moment to herself in case she broke down in front of both Harvey and her family and told them exactly what had happened in Fiji. She'd almost spluttered when Brody had asked about wild nights, because there had been plenty of those. As for broken hearts, she'd naively assumed hers was untouchable, but Harvey had found a way to get under her guard, to make her fall for him, until she'd become the cliché she'd mocked other women for: past her expiration date, but left wanting more. So much more.

She'd stupidly fallen in love with Harvey, a man who couldn't love her back because he'd spent years shutting down his emotions and feeling unworthy of love. And that wasn't all. That morning, before leaving Auckland for Melbourne, she'd taken a pregnancy test, discovering she was pregnant.

Locking herself in the bathroom now, Della rested her hand on her stomach, choked with happiness. She was finally achieving one of her dreams. A baby. Harvey's baby. But it changed nothing. Of course she needed to tell him, and soon. How would he take the news? Would he be angry? Feel trapped? She had no doubt that he cared for Della and that, in time, he'd do right by their child. But that wasn't how she'd envisioned having a family. She wanted to be in love and loved in return.

She wanted to build a home with that love of her life. She wanted forever.

Della blinked away the sting in her eyes. Harvey had urged her to be uncompromising when it came to her dreams and desires, to reach for it all and never settle. Of course he couldn't have known that he'd become tangled up in those dreams. That she'd want to spend the rest of her life with *him*, have *his* baby. But Della couldn't make him feel something for her that he just wasn't capable of. Better to take what was on offer, his friendship and respect. Better for them to focus on being parents, separate but united for their child. This time, it was better to strategically settle than to risk losing a chunk of her heart she wasn't sure she'd survive without.

While she washed her hands, she splashed cold water on her face and avoided looking at her reflection in the mirror. She knew what she'd see. A woman in love. A woman who in fact, despite all her tough talk and Harvey's encouragement, *couldn't* have it all. A woman who'd made another mistake and fallen for a broken man incapable of loving her back. Because to Harvey, love was weakness. Powerlessness. A price too high.

Della emerged from the bathroom, reluctant to head back outside just yet. Distracted by the framed photographs lining the hallway, she took a closer look. She'd never really noticed them before, but they were pictures of Harvey with all the important people in his life. One of him and Brody in their twenties, dressed in tuxedos at some medic's ball. One of Harvey and Bill dressed in hiking gear on the top of Victoria's Mount Oberon. One of Christmas at the Wiltons', everyone wearing paper hats as they raised a toast to the camera.

Her family was Harvey's too. He loved them and they him. All the more reason for Della to tread with caution so neither of them lost what they valued. She spied herself in the last photo, struggling to identify which Christmas it was. But even then, all those years ago, some part of her had wanted Harvey, had been halfway in love with him. She would likely always have unresolved feelings for Harvey. But she'd survive that. What she wouldn't survive was loving him with her whole heart when he didn't love her bàck.

Della was just about to turn away, to head to the garden and tell her family she was calling it a night, when a pair of hands gripped her waist. 'There you are. I've been trying to get you alone all night.'

His warm breath tickled the side of her neck and she shuddered, his touch sparking her body alive as if she'd been in a coma for two long weeks. Della turned, bracing herself against how handsome he was, how it physically hurt to look at him because he could never be hers. His eyes danced with the excitement she'd waited two endless weeks to see.

'Come with me,' he said. She meekly followed, clinging to his hand as he tugged her into a nearby room, which turned out to be his home office.

He shut the door and pulled her into his arms. The force of wanting him almost buckled her knees, but panic beat at her ribs.

'Shouldn't we head back outside before they come looking for us?' she said feebly as he cupped her face and slid his fingers into her hair, tilting up her chin.

'Brody's taken Amy and Jack home,' he breathed against her lips. 'I think both your parents have dozed off sitting around the fire pit.' Without another word, he pressed his lips to hers and just let them sit there for a handful of seconds as he breathed in deeply. Della sighed, sagged against him, her entire body melting as if she was finally home. But he couldn't be her safe place. She needed to be strong for their baby and for her own stupid heart.

'God, I've missed you,' he said, pulling back to stare deep into her eyes.

Della saw longing and desire and euphoria in the depths of his eyes, but it still wasn't enough. She wanted more of him. She wanted all of him—the good and the bad and the broken. She wanted impossible things.

'Why didn't you tell me when you were arriving?' he said, wrapping his arms around her shoulders so her head rested on his chest. 'I'd have picked you up from the airport.'

Della shrugged, her heart so sore she could barely breathe. 'You were busy here, and how would we have explained that to the others?'

Harvey stiffened, rested his hands on her shoulders and peeled her away so he could look at her. 'Is everything okay? You've been avoiding me all night. I've been going out of my mind. I wanted to kiss you so badly.'

'I thought the plan was to play it cool,' Della lied. She'd ignored him because to be close to him was torture. Because she'd almost snapped so many times tonight and confessed that she loved him. Because the part of her that yet again had realised too late she'd have to compromise her dreams wanted him anyway, as she'd known she would.

Della swallowed, stepping back but wishing she was

still in his arms, where things made a twisted kind of sense. 'We don't need Brody and his intrusive questions. I swear Amy is a saint for putting up with my brother.'

'Can you stay?' he asked, reaching for her again. 'Here. With me, tonight? After everyone else leaves.'

Della rested her hand on his chest, felt the rapid pound of his heart, wished that it beat with love for her. 'I can't... We agreed.' Her throat ached with longing. Why had she ever thought she could be this man's friend? She'd known it had been impossible the first time she'd met him. Now, twenty years later, when she knew him better than ever, there was no hope. She loved him. She craved him. She wanted him. *Friends* was for the runner-up.

'Della... I've been thinking,' he said when she stayed silent, because she was desperately trying not to cry. 'I've missed you so badly since I arrived home.'

'Me too,' she said, her throat tight. She refused to cry. She didn't want to blurt out her irrelevant feelings or her news about the baby. She'd planned it all on the flight. She'd tell him tomorrow, after Jack's naming day party.

He smiled, and her heart cracked a little more. 'I really want you to apply for the job in my department. Us working together has to be better than this—missing each other, waking up alone, not to mention the abstinence.' He shot her a playful smile that two weeks ago she could have returned. But not now.

'I... I'm not sure, Harvey.' Della shook her head, looked down. She wanted more than sex. She wanted it all. She always had. The only change was that she wanted it with him—Harvey Ward.

'I know it's complicated,' Harvey rushed on, 'and I don't have the first clue what I'm doing, but if you move back here, maybe we could, you know, try dating. Each other, I mean.' He exhaled a sigh, as if speaking those words had left him exhausted.

Della's chest ached. Of course he would struggle with dating, but she could see how hard he was trying. That he genuinely meant what he'd said. That the first tentative step towards a relationship was a huge step for Harvey. But they'd always been too different when it came to commitment, and that hadn't changed. Della was miles ahead, a place where she was sure to get hurt. And what then? What about the baby?

'You know I haven't done this in a very long time,' he continued, misinterpreting her hesitance. 'I know I'm a risk, but it could work. *We* could work.' Before she could reply, he hauled her close, bringing her lips up to his, sliding his tongue against hers, filling her body with love hormones. Della surrendered, luxuriating in his kisses, which, after two parched weeks in the desert, felt like heaven. But the high faltered, her head intruding. She'd have to turn him down. She'd have to tell him why.

Because she was too scared to part with her secret just yet, because she wanted him, one last time, in spite of how ridiculously out of sync they were when it came to relationships, Della allowed herself the indulgence of his strong arms, his frantic kisses, the hot possessive surge of his tongue against hers. Oh, how she'd missed him, the breadth of his smile and the playful glint in his eyes. The feel of his strong arms and the beat of his heart. The way he believed in her and the way he made her feel. She panted, preparing to stop this. To walk away before any more of her heart was eroded, but her fingers flexed in his shirt, her head falling back so he could ravage her neck, her moans encouraging.

'That was the worst two weeks of my life,' he said, hoisting her onto the desk. One of his thighs slotted between her legs as he pressed kisses over her face, her neck, the tops of her breasts and back to her lips. 'Every day I wanted to call you. The only reason I didn't call was to give you the space you wanted, to pretend that we could be friends. But it's not working for me.'

As his lips parted hers once more, his hand cupped her breast through her dress. Pregnancy hormones had made her sensitive, but his touch set her alight, inflamed her from head to toe. She twisted his hair in her fingers and rubbed the hard length of him through his shorts. Just one more time... Then, at the end of the weekend, she'd tell him about the baby and fly back to Auckland, where she could patch up her bruised heart away from this temptation.

Reaching for his fly, she dragged her kiss-swollen lips from his. 'Hurry,' she said, 'I want you.' If this was the only part of him she could have, she'd take it and worry about the price later.

Harvey didn't argue. While she undid his shorts and pushed them over his hips, taking him in her hand, he lifted her dress and shoved her underwear down her legs, his tongue in her mouth.

Della spread her thighs, making room for his hips, casting the closed office door a nervous glance. But she was too far gone to care about interruptions, too high on the decadence of Harvey's touch to voice caution. Too lovesick to protect her battle-worn heart. She would love him with her body, silently say goodbye. Then she'd walk away from one dream and focus on being the best parent she could be.

Dragging his mouth from hers, Harvey dropped to his knees, shoving her dress up her thighs. 'I locked the door,' he said before covering her with his mouth.

Della closed her eyes against the intense wave of pleasure. Dizzy with it, she braced one hand on the desk behind her and tunnelled the other into Harvey's hair, holding on for dear life.

'Harvey,' she gasped, looking down at him. His eyes were dark with desire and determination, his hands on her thighs, gripping her tight. Pleasure built and built, the sharp ache only a fraction of the pain she'd endured these two weeks without him. But she couldn't keep him. She had to put the baby first. Put herself first.

Her moans grew. She released Harvey's hair and covered her mouth, bit the back of her hand to hold them inside. As if he knew her body, knew how close she was, Harvey jerked to his feet, gripped her hips and slowly pushed inside her. Della clung to his shoulders, wrapped her legs around his hips and dragged his mouth down to hers. Harvey bucked into her, his pace as frantic as the beat of her heart, his kisses as deep as his possession of her body, his passion for her almost enough to make her change her mind. Almost.

Della wanted more than passion. More than really great sex. She wanted him to love her as desperately as she loved him. She wanted them to raise their baby together in that house with the clichéd white picket fence. She wanted him to feel the terrifying fear and powerlessness of love and want it anyway, with *her*. But those dreams belonged to Della, not to Harvey.

Her orgasm ripped through her, and she sobbed his name. Harvey crushed her in his arms and groaned, joining her, his fingers and his whispers in her hair.

'I missed you,' he said, his breath see-sawing in his chest. 'I missed you so much.'

Della hid her face against his neck, blinking the sting of tears from her eyes. That had been a big mistake. 'I'd better go before my parents come looking for one of us.' She pushed him away, slid from the desk and scooped up her underwear from the floor. She needed to get away from him before she begged him to love her.

'You're leaving?' he said, confusion clouding his handsome face as he tucked himself back into his shorts. 'Just hang around until they leave. Stay the night. I'll make you breakfast, and we can go to Jack's thing together.'

'I can't, Harvey. I—' she broke off, realisation dawning. She couldn't wait any longer. She had to tell him now. He deserved to know about the baby, and her confession, the knowledge that he was going to be a father, would put everything back into perspective for him the way it had for Della that morning. She wanted him like oxygen, but this was no longer just about her desires.

'Did you see the job's been advertised?' he pressed, a desperate look in his eyes. 'You should apply. They need someone to start as soon as possible.'

'Harvey, we need to talk.' She straightened her dress and folded her arms across her waist, holding her fractured pieces together.

'Okay, come and have a drink. Perhaps your parents have already left.'

Della shook her head. 'No. I don't want a drink. I just want you to listen.' Just like they had when they'd left

Fiji, it was better to make a clean break of it now. The sex was over, as great as it had been. Now there were bigger issues to work on than if they should be colleagues or whether or not they could make a relationship work.

'Okay. I'm listening.' He reached for her hand, and she paced away. If he touched her again, she'd mess this up, say the wrong things, beg him to love her or worse, settle for only a part of him, not the whole.

'I didn't want to tell you until tomorrow, after the party,' she began, a chill spreading along her bare arms, 'but I'm pregnant, Harvey.' She looked up, saw the flash of disbelief in his eyes and rushed on. 'We made a baby in Fiji. Probably that time in the waterfall.'

Confusion shifted in his stare. He opened his mouth to speak. Closed it again. Shook his head, as dumbfounded as she'd been that morning, seeing those two pink lines.

'I know I reassured you that I was on the pill,' she rushed on, 'which I was. But obviously I must have missed one or something. And I know that you never wanted kids. I know this—' she placed her hand on her stomach '—is my dream, not yours. But I want you to know that you don't have to feel responsible. You don't have to do anything or say anything or be anything you're not ready to be. I understand.'

Poor Harvey. He'd only just decided that he might want a relationship, and now he was going to be a father. Talk about life in fast forward... At his bewilderment, she winced, hating herself for her lack of willpower. If she hadn't slept with him again, maybe she could have kept her secret until a more appropriate time. 'I know it's a lot to take in. You're probably angry and upset—'

'I'm not angry,' he said, his jaw clenched as he

scrubbed a hand through his hair, glancing down at her flat stomach. 'Are you...okay?'

Della nodded, brushing aside his concern. If he carried on being wonderful and thoughtful, she was going to cry. As it was, this baby would probably be born holding a box of tissues, she'd cried so much over Harvey this past fortnight.

'Obviously this weekend is about Amy and Brody and baby Jack,' she said, also reminding herself that she couldn't be properly excited yet and tell anyone else. 'I know we'll need to explain about us eventually, but I think it's best if we keep this to ourselves for now and figure everything else out later. I'll, um...call you from Auckland, and we can talk everything through.'

Harvey's frown deepened, his helpless expression hardening. 'Wait,' he said, stepping forward and reaching for her arm.

Della stepped back, ducked out of his reach. She couldn't let him touch her again or she'd break down.

'You're going back to Auckland?' he asked, incredulous, his stare carrying pain and accusation.

Nausea swirled in her stomach. 'Of course, Harvey. I live there. My home is there. My job.' She couldn't just drop everything. She needed time to think.

'So you're not going to apply for the job here?' He gripped the back of his neck and paced back and forth. 'Where we could raise our baby together?'

A wild flutter of hope bloomed in her chest. Could she do that? Move home, work with Harvey, have his baby and hope that in time, he might fall in love with her? Could she settle for so little when she wanted it all? If it worked, it would be everything she'd ever dreamed. But if it failed, would she survive? Maybe if she hadn't fallen in love with him, she could return and just see what happened. But it was too late for what-ifs.

'I'm not sure yet,' she whispered, fear and guilt and loathing forcing her stare from his. 'I'll certainly think about the job. But like you, I'm in shock. I only found out about the baby myself this morning, and now I have to think about things like maternity leave...' Della swallowed hard, wishing dreams were that easy. She knew from experience that reaching for it all, pinning her hopes on a man who wasn't sure what he wanted, could backfire. She couldn't make that mistake again, not when there was their baby to consider. She needed to trust her instincts.

He came to a standstill and stared her way. 'So, if you're not sure about the job, you're even less sure about me, about us having a relationship? And yet you let me prattle on about dating, knowing you were going to turn me down.'

Della pressed her lips together, her throat raw with emotion. 'I'm sorry. I wasn't thinking straight.' Had she selfishly used him again? 'I just know that I need to put the baby first. *We* need to put the baby first. This isn't about us anymore, and you and I still want different things.' Dating wasn't enough, not when she loved him so desperately. She'd overreached before, pushed for more and lost. It was better to forget about love and focus on the baby.

'I get it.' Harvey nodded, his stare bleak. 'I'm fine as a sperm donor, I'm fine for sex, but I'm just not up to scratch when it comes to relationships.'

'I didn't say that,' she said, looking away from the pain

in his eyes. 'I want us to do this, the baby, together. I just haven't figured out all the details yet.'

'It's okay. I understand,' Harvey said, heading for the door. 'You'll have my baby, but good old Harvey couldn't possibly be anything serious, least of all a husband, right, not when there's probably a better option out there somewhere?'

He left the room, left Della with the echo of his pain and resentment. Rather than face her parents, rather than hurt herself or Harvey any more tonight, Della slipped out of the front door and escaped.

CHAPTER FOURTEEN

HARVEY PRESSED HIS lips to the top of Jack's head and breathed in his clean baby smell, his stare glued to the door of the party venue for a first glimpse of Della. He'd arrived early at the trendy restaurant near Brody and Amy's suburb, which had a small function room for events. His house was too big and too quiet now that he knew not only that he was going to be a father, but that Della wanted nothing more to do with him beyond some depressing shared custody arrangement.

She'd rejected him, as much as told him he wasn't good enough for her to risk her heart, that she could never love a man like him. And he couldn't even be angry, because maybe she was right.

'Are you nervous?' Brody asked, reaching for his son.

Nervous? He was bereft. Della might as well have ripped his heart out of his chest last night and looked down on it with disappointment. He wasn't enough for her, even after everything they'd shared, even when he'd offered to give her everything he could, even when they'd made a child together.

'I'm not nervous,' he reassured Brody, chilled to the bone, because he was so gutted by her rejection he couldn't even be properly excited by the news of his baby.

'I'll be fine.' If *fine* meant desolate, inadequate, helpless like never before.

'The others are risking being late,' Brody said about Della and Mr and Mrs W, looking slightly harassed. He bounced on the balls of his feet to keep the baby happy.

'Should I call Della?' Harvey asked, tension tightening his shoulders. 'Find out where they are?' Maybe they were having car trouble. Maybe Della was ill or there was something wrong with the baby. He'd give her two more minutes, and then he was going to look for her.

Brody scoffed, handing the baby his phone to stop him fussing. 'You calling her would only make her grumpy. We don't want bickering today of all days.'

Harvey rubbed a hand down his face in frustration. Was his friend truly that blind? Why had he never noticed the way Harvey felt about Della? The way he'd *always* felt? Was Harvey that good at hiding his feelings? Because now, when it was over between them, when he'd finally realised that he'd fallen deeply in love with Della in Fiji, he could finally admit that those feelings had always run deep inside him, waiting for the timing to be right. Except nothing was right without Della.

'Haven't you ever stopped to wonder why Della and I are always at each other's throats?' he snapped, taking his frustration out on his clueless friend.

Brody shrugged, distracted. 'You're just too different, that's all.'

'That's not all.' He couldn't do it any longer, pretend that he wasn't crazy about her, that he just wanted sex or friendship or some depressing co-parenting situation. He wanted Della. 'This might be hard for you hear,' he said, past the point of no return, 'but I've always fancied your sister.'

Brody looked up, startled.

'When I first met her,' Harvey continued, 'I was in such a bad place, I knew I couldn't act on it without hurting her or messing up our friendship.'

'My sister?' Brody gaped in disbelief.

Harvey nodded and gripped the back of his neck, his panic mounting. 'I'm in love with her,' he said in a rush. '*She's* the one I care about. *She's* the reason everything has changed for me.' *She* was worth this sickening feeling of fear and inadequacy that made him feel eight years old again.

Brody's eyebrows shot up, and then a slow grin spread over his face. 'Harvey Ward finally falling in love, and it's for my little sister?'

Harvey shook his head and paced away in disgust. 'I shouldn't have told you,' he muttered foully. This was serious. He loved her and he'd lost her because she couldn't believe in him, couldn't want him, couldn't choose him.

'Don't be like that,' Brody said, sobering. 'Does she love you too?'

Harvey shot his friend an incredulous look. 'Don't be stupid. She's an intelligent woman. She could never take me seriously, and she's probably right not to. I don't know the first thing about committed relationships. And I don't want to let her down or hurt her. She's been through enough.' Della was scared, too. Scared to trust her instincts, scared to be hurt again, scared to want her dreams. Why would she take a chance on a beginner like him, especially now that they had their baby to consider? But he'd keep that part of the story to himself for now.

'That bickering you two always do, you know that's two-sided, right?' Brody said, as if he'd completely missed the point Harvey was trying to make.

'Yeah, so?' Harvey checked the time, frantic now for Della to arrive so he could ensure she was okay.

'Duh…' Brody said, as if reverting to a teenager. 'Della's always had a bit of thing for you. I used to tease her about it. I never told you, obviously, because…you know…she's my sister.'

Harvey shook his head, in no way comforted. Just because she'd always fancied him, just because they were great together physically, didn't mean she was ready to trust him, of all men, with her massive heart. She wasn't even ready to be his colleague, to raise their baby with him, to give him a chance to forge a proper relationship. She didn't want him, and there was nothing he could do to change that.

'It doesn't matter,' Harvey said, too heartsore to explain the details. 'She wants us to be friends.' To raise their baby together but nothing more.

Brody frowned, sceptically, realisation seeming to dawn. 'You haven't told her, have you? That you're in love with her.'

Harvey winced, his chest too small for his lungs. 'I tried…last night…' But he hadn't been able to get the words out. A part of him, the part that had shut down any emotional connection for the past twenty years, still worried he was unworthy of love, especially the love of a woman as amazing as Della.

'Seriously?' Brody asked, inching closer and lowering his voice. 'Don't try, just tell her.'

Harvey curled his hands into fists. Would she care

when she'd already decided a relationship with him wasn't enough? Was he setting himself up for another slap of rejection if he told her his true feelings? Was he at risk of not just losing Della, but also of their chance to be parents who got along and respected each other?

'Don't be stupid, man,' Brody pressed. 'She's flying back to Auckland tonight. If you don't tell her today, you might regret it.'

Harvey nodded numbly, his brain firing normally for the first time this weekend. Of course he would regret it. He loved Della, and she needed to know. Even if she could never take him seriously or love him back, he should tell her how she'd made him believe in love again.

'I'm going to find her,' he said, heading for the exit without waiting for permission.

'Don't be late,' Brody called after him. 'My son is counting on you.'

Graham Wilton pulled into the last available parking space outside the restaurant where Jack's naming day party was taking place and turned off the engine.

Della's stomach lurched with despair and anguish. How would she face Harvey today and not completely break down? She'd hurt him last night. Thrown his offer of dating back in his face. Rejected him, just like his mother.

'Can you give us a moment, darling?' Della's mother said to her husband from the passenger seat. 'I just need a word with Della.'

Della shifted in the back seat of the car, checking her watch. 'We're cutting it pretty fine, Mum.' The last thing she needed when she was feeling so bereft was her mum digging around in Della's head.

'This won't take long,' Jenny said, popping her seat belt and turning to face her daughter. 'Especially if you just come out and tell me what's wrong instead of denying it.'

Della sighed, glancing down at her hands twisting in her lap. Of course her mother would pick up on her mood. 'Nothing's wrong,' she started, scared that if she began the story, she'd cry and ruin Jack's photos with her blotchy red face. She looked up, met her mother's sympathetic stare. 'I'm pregnant, that's all.'

Jenny's hand gripped Della's. 'That's wonderful news. I'm so happy for you. Are you feeling okay?'

Della nodded robotically. 'I'm fine. It's very early. Obviously it's Jack's day, and I don't want to tell anyone else yet.'

Jenny nodded, her astute expression turning curious. 'Who's the father?'

Della dragged in a deep breath. This was the tricky part. The risk of breaking down and confessing to her mother that she'd stupidly fallen in love with Harvey Ward. 'It's Harvey.'

Her mother's eyes widened. 'Our Harvey?'

'Of course, Mum. I don't know any other Harveys.' Now that she'd told him her news, now that she'd protected her heart and put the baby first, now that she'd relied on her instincts and refused to settle for less than she deserved, she was supposed to feel better. But if anything, she felt worse. She'd barely slept a wink last night, replaying that last conversation over and over until nothing made sense. Reliving the hurt in Harvey's eyes. The rejection and the heartbreaking acceptance, as if he'd been expecting it all along.

'Oh, my…' Jenny said, with a flash of respect. 'I didn't know you two were—'

'We're not,' Della said flatly. 'It happened in Fiji.'

Jenny nodded, knowingly. 'Of course. Well, he's always liked you.'

Della looked up, her heart withering a little more. If only he could do more than like her. If only he wanted more than a *try it and see* relationship. If only he could love her. 'Yes, well, I just want to get through today, so if you could not mention it to Dad or Brody or Amy, and maybe stop looking at me like that.'

'Like what?' Jenny asked innocently. 'Like I'm about to ask what your plans are?'

'Exactly.' Della sighed as Jenny waited for her to elaborate. 'My plan is to go back to New Zealand and have a good long think,' she said, caving to pressure. 'My plan is to focus on raising my baby, with as much input from Harvey as he wants, obviously.'

'And what about you and Harvey?' Jenny asked, a flicker of sympathy in her eyes. 'What about having a relationship?'

'Come on, Mum. This is Harvey,' Della said, glancing out of the car window to stop herself from crying. 'He's not really ready for a relationship, not that I can blame him. But the most important thing for all of us, him, me and the baby, is if we're…friends.'

Jenny frowned, her eyes full of questions. 'But you're in love with him.'

'I am.' The admission should have filled her with joy.

'How is that going to factor into your *friendship*?'

Della ducked her head in shame. 'Obviously it's not. I'll get over it. I'll put the baby first, and I'll be fine.'

Jenny nodded in agreement. 'Yes, you will. But you won't have everything you've ever wanted. Does Harvey know that you're in love with him? Have you told him how you feel? Because if you really love him, it's not just going to go away, and he deserves to know something so important.'

Della shook her head, her eyes burning. 'No. I... I didn't think it was relevant. We still want different things.'

Except what had Harvey meant when he'd said 'good old Harvey couldn't possibly be anything serious, least of all a husband'?

'Harvey thinks he wants to try and have a relationship,' she went on, more confused than ever, 'but I can't be his trial run, putting my feelings on hold, loving him but waiting around to see if a relationship is what he genuinely wants. I just can't.' It would destroy her.

'But if you haven't told him how you feel and what *you* want, you haven't really given him a chance to step up, have you?' Jenny tilted her head, seeing way too much for Della's liking. 'What if he needs to know that you love him? What if he loves you too?'

Della glared, her heart in her throat. Of course, Harvey needed to be loved as much as the next person, perhaps more so after everything he'd been through. She shook her head even as hope rushed through her like an electrical storm. 'He can't love me. He's spent most of his adult life shutting down, keeping people out.'

Jenny smiled sadly. 'And you're still scared to want it all in case you make another mistake.'

Della swallowed, sick to her stomach. Had she written

Harvey off too soon, because she was still scared to trust her judgement, still settling for less than she deserved? Still terrified to reach for all of her dreams? Had she unfairly judged him, rejected him the way his mother had, when in reality, she loved and wanted every inch of him, even if he didn't love her back?

'You've always been scared to fail,' Jenny said, squeezing Della's fingers. 'I blame myself and your father. We inadvertently created a very competitive household. But your drive is your strength. Don't let one relationship failure hold you back from having everything you want. Tell Harvey how you feel and give him a chance.'

Della nodded numbly, feeling stupid. A small, building sense of panic was choking her. Her mother was right.

'Come on,' Jenny said, opening the passenger side door. 'We'd better go inside. The ceremony is about to start.'

Della slammed the car door and rushed inside the venue. Was she too late to undo the damage she'd inflicted last night when she'd hurt both Harvey and herself with her fear? Her mother was right. Harvey deserved to know that she loved him, even if he couldn't return her feelings. To know that, of all men, Della chose *him*.

CHAPTER FIFTEEN

HARVEY HADN'T MADE it to Della in time. Just as she and her mother had walked into the room, her eyes meeting his for an electrifying beat, the celebrant had announced it was time to start. All throughout the naming day ceremony, as together they'd promised to guide and support Jack, he'd struggled to take his eyes off her. She looked beautiful, her simple blue dress matching the colour of her eyes, and her hair casually pinned up to expose her neck. It had been torture fighting the urge to drag her aside and tell her how he felt about her, but somehow he'd managed to put Brody, Amy and Jack first temporarily.

Outside in the garden at the side of the restaurant, Harvey's cheek muscles twitched from the pressure of maintaining a semi-fake smile. But he didn't want to ruin Jack's photos.

'And one last smile, please,' the photographer said, snapping the final photo—Amy and Brody in the centre holding Jack with Harvey and Della at either end.

The minute the photographer checked the shot in the digital display, Harvey moved to intercept Della, panic like ice in his veins. But his patience had run out.

'Della, we need to talk,' he said as Amy and Brody wandered back inside with Jack.

'Yes, of course, we do,' she said, blinking up at him. 'Harvey, I'm so sorry about last night.' She reached for his arm. 'I was all over the place. I'd like to blame my hormones, but I think that would be a lie.'

Harvey shook his head, cutting her off, drawing her deeper into the shade of a tree out of the sun. 'No. *I'm* sorry.' He took her hand from his arm and squeezed her fingers. 'I was stupid, Della. I was so excited to see you after these past two weeks that I stepped in my own way, and I forgot to tell you the most important thing.'

He gripped her arms, wishing they were somewhere more romantic than a garden so he could convince her that he meant what he was about to say. But he'd just have to risk that this, here and now, would be enough. 'I love you, Della. I fell in love with you in Fiji, and I should have told you as soon as I realised.'

She blinked, her eyes wide with confusion and doubt.

'I was scared,' he rushed on, his hands skimming her upper arms, because he couldn't not touch her. 'Scared that I'm not enough for you, because I'm a forty-two-year-old man who's never been in love before, not like this.' He pressed a fist to the centre of his chest, where it burned the most. 'Scared that you deserve someone better at relationships. That if I tried to be what you need, I'd fail and let you down, and I never want to be a man who lets you down.' He shook his head, the idea abhorrent.

'Harvey...' she whispered, her eyes shining with un-shed tears. 'You *are* enough.'

But the pressure to say what he should have said last night was overwhelming. He slid his hands down her bare arms and gripped her fingers. 'I know I'm a big risk for you, and I know that you're scared. I know that we wanted different things in the past, and that you've been hurt and let down before. I know that we can't afford to mess this up, because we're already a massive part of each other's lives. But I've half loved you for twenty years, Della. I was just too scared to fall all the way in case I discovered that there was, in fact, something unlovable about me. Something that meant you could never choose me.'

Della shook her head, tears landing on her cheeks. 'No, there isn't, and I do.'

'But I'm not scared anymore,' he said, only half hearing her as he cupped her face and wiped a tear away with the pad of his thumb. 'Well, that's not strictly true. I *am* scared. I'm terrified. But mainly about losing you, or having to live without you. So if you'll just give me a chance, one chance, at our relationship, I promise that I'll try and give you everything you've ever wanted. I'll try every day to be what you deserve. I'll never stop trying to make us work, because I'll always love you.'

Della laughed through her tears, throwing her arms around his neck. 'Harvey, you are already everything I want. You, us, the baby.'

'Really?' he asked, the lump in his throat so big he thought he might choke. But he was smart enough to grip her tight in case she changed her mind.

Della nodded, standing on her toes to press her lips to his. 'I'm sorry that I made you doubt yourself. It wasn't that you weren't enough. It was that *I* was still scared to trust my instincts and go after all of my dreams. But you showed me that I didn't have to settle, that I can have it all, as long as I follow my heart. And my heart leads to you, Harvey. I love you, too.'

Harvey held her close, his heart thudding wildly. 'Don't

say it if you don't mean it,' he choked out, overcome. He was willing to hold on to her forever in the hopes that one day she might love him in return. As long as it took.

'I do mean it,' she cried, cupping his face. 'I want to move back to Melbourne and work with you, and raise our baby with you, and grow old with you, although I can't promise that we won't bicker from time to time.'

Harvey grinned, his heart soaring with hope. 'What's a little bit of harmless bickering when we're so good together in all other areas?' Before she could answer, he hauled her into his arms and slanted his lips over hers, kissing her with everything he was. Their tongues glided together, her fingers twisting his hair as her body shifted restlessly against his, seeking more.

Harvey pulled back, panting hard, her face gripped between his palms. 'You really love me?'

She leaned back and looked up at him, her emotions shining in her eyes. 'Of course I do. I almost told you last night, but then I thought you couldn't love me, and so I left first. I sabotaged this before you could hurt me, but I'm done being scared. I'm done putting my dreams on hold. I want us to build a life together. I want it all, and I know you can be everything I need, because you already are. I choose you, Harvey.'

Dragging her close again, Harvey kissed her until his head swam from lack of oxygen. 'Can we get out of here yet?' he asked, drying the rest of her tears. 'I want to take you home to bed before you fly back to New Zealand.'

Della laughed, rubbing at her smudged mascara. 'I think my brother might never speak to us again if we did that.'

Harvey shrugged, willing to risk it if she was, but they

owed it to Jack to be present, not that the cute little fella would ever remember their sacrifice.

Della sobered, searching his stare. 'How do you feel… about the baby?' she asked with a frown of concern. 'I know it wasn't planned, and you're going from being alone to being in a relationship *and* being a father. That's a lot.'

His hands held her waist, but he wanted to drop to his knees and press a kiss to her stomach, where their baby grew. 'I feel like the luckiest man alive, Della. I love kids—tiny cute humans. I always have. They were just something else I denied myself because I was so used to holding back my emotions. But I don't know, something happened in Fiji. I kept seeing a different side to you and then another and then another, and I found myself helpless to letting you in. I found myself telling you things I've never told anyone else.'

She nodded. 'Me too.'

'But how are *you* feeling? Any morning sickness? You look a little tired?' Guilt for the way they'd left things last night crawled over his skin.

'I'm okay. I didn't sleep well last night,' she said, pressing her lips to his with a breathy sigh. 'But it's my own fault. I met this gorgeous man in Fiji and had the best sex of my life, the best holiday fling, and then I fell in love. But when I saw him again, I bottled it, despite being crazy about him, despite choosing him of all men.'

Harvey grinned, his ego inflating. 'The best sex, huh? Tell me more.'

Della rolled her eyes. 'Of course that's the thing you focus on.'

Laughing, he wrapped his arm around her shoulders

and pressed a kiss to her temple as they headed back inside to the party. 'That first day in Fiji, you said it wasn't that great, so I'm just clarifying the details.'

Della nudged him with her elbow, tilting her face up for another kiss. 'Don't gloat.'

'I'm afraid you can't stop me.' He paused in the doorway and cupped her face, brushing his lips over hers.

When he pulled back, she looked up at him, slipping her arm around his waist, her other hand gripping his fingers on her shoulder. 'What will we tell them about us?'

She meant her family, the Wiltons, and Bill too, who'd been invited to join the celebration. Harvey smiled, never more certain of anything in his life than he was about Della. 'We'll tell them the truth. We'll tell them I fell in love with you in Fiji.'

Della shook her head, that familiar spark of challenge he loved in her eyes. 'No, we'll tell them *I* fell in love with *you*.'

'Okay, you win.' He winked, chasing her lips with his in a final kiss before they pushed open the door to the restaurant and stepped into their future.

EPILOGUE

Two years later.

DELLA'S PAGER SOUNDED, summoning her to theatre. Her next patient must have left the surgical ward. She silenced the device, which was clipped to the pocket of her green Melbourne Medical Centre scrubs, and took the stairs. She was just about to turn the corner into the operating suites when Australia's hottest surgeon appeared in her path.

'Well, fancy meeting you here, Dr Wilton,' Harvey said, his stare travelling her body with a look that was way too indecent for the workplace.

'Are you following me again, Dr Ward?' she said, her breath trapped in her chest at how handsome he was and how, after almost two years of marriage, she was still crazy in love with him. 'Because you seem to be everywhere I look—in *my* bed, at *my* work, father to *my* children.' Pointedly, she glanced down at her pregnant belly, resting a hand over their growing son. 'If I didn't know you better, I'd guess you were my husband or something.'

They'd married in an intimate ceremony with family and friends four months before the birth of baby Lily, their daughter.

Harvey grinned, glanced along the corridor and then opened the nearest door, dragging Della into a utility room, the shelves of which were stacked with folded clean bed linens. 'Man, I missed you,' he said, hauling her as close as the baby bump would allow.

Della kissed him back, finally pulling back with a chuckle. 'Since this morning?'

'Yes,' he said simply, his expression sincere. That playful glint came into his eyes, doubling Della's pulse. 'Believe it or not, being married to you is the best thing that's ever happened to this old reformed bachelor. And the sex…' He rolled his eyes closed and groaned. 'Don't even get me started on how good that is. Some might say the best of their life…?'

Della laughed, too happy with his smug confidence to pull him up on his arrogance. When it came to accepting her love, trusting in it and giving her everything in return, her husband had risen to the top of the class during the past two years.

'I have to go,' she said, kissing him swiftly once more. 'I have a man who came off his motorbike yesterday about to arrive in theatre.'

Harvey gripped her waist, blocking her escape. 'One more kiss to get me through the afternoon,' he begged, sliding his lips up the side of her neck so she shuddered against him with desire.

As she did every day, Della tangled her fingers in his hair and kissed him properly—her lips parting, her tongue sliding against his, her body shifting restlessly as she tried to manage how much he turned her on.

'Wow,' Harvey said when they parted, looking a little dazed. 'That was some kiss.'

'I'm softening you up,' she said, running her fingers through his hair in order to make him look presentable for his patients. 'Do you want day care pickup or dinner?'

Harvey groaned half-heartedly. 'Come on… I made dinner last night.'

'Perhaps you prefer both,' she said, playfully digging in her heels. 'My surgery will probably run over anyway.'

'Fine,' he said with a mock sigh, 'I suppose I'll pick up my adorable daughter from nursery and make my pregnant wife a delicious, nutritious meal for when she gets home from work.' Finally turning serious, he cupped her face and kissed her one last time. 'Leave it to me—the best sex and the best husband you've ever had.'

Della laughed, loving his competitive streak as much as she loved the rest of him. 'Don't forget the best father to our children,' she said, reaching for the door handle. Just before she left the glorified cupboard to sheepishly make her exit, hoping no one would see, she turned back. 'I love you.'

She never tired of saying that to Harvey. Nor had she ever grown used to the hint of bewilderment she saw in his eyes every time she did, as if he couldn't quite believe it was true.

'I love you too, Della.' He reached for her hand and squeezed her fingers. 'See you at home.'

She opened the door and was about to duck out when he pulled her back. His lips found hers, his hands gripping her face so tight, she forgot to breathe as he kissed her. When he pulled back, he rested his forehead against hers and whispered, 'Do you have everything that you've ever wanted?'

Dazed from the passion and desperation of his kiss and
awash with love hormones, Della nodded, lost for words.
'Good,' Harvey said. 'Because that makes two of us.'

* * * * *

If you enjoyed this story,
check out these other great reads from
JC Harroway

Secretly Dating the Baby Doc
Nurse's Secret Royal Fling
Her Secret Valentine's Baby
Phoebe's Baby Bombshell

All available now!

COMING SOON!

We really hope you enjoyed reading this book.
If you're looking for more romance
be sure to head to the shops when
new books are available on

Thursday 21st November

To see which titles are coming soon, please visit
millsandboon.co.uk/nextmonth

MILLS & BOON

MILLS & BOON®

Coming next month

MELTING DR GRUMPY'S FROZEN HEART
Scarlet Wilson

This guy didn't know her background. He didn't know why she was here.

For Skye, cancer research was personal. But she didn't know his background, or what had made him do years of training and decide that oncology was the place he wanted to work. She wasn't here to make an enemy. But from the expression on his face, she was doubting she was making a friend.

She decided to push in another direction. 'You know,' she said breezily, 'I am a huge Christmas fan. You'll learn that over the next few weeks. My favourite movie is The Grinch. I'd hate for people to start calling you that.'

The edges of his mouth hinted upwards and he gave a sigh, as his eyebrows raised. The expression had the hint of a cheeky teenager about it. 'My nickname is Dr Grumpy, and yes, I know that,' he replied in that delicious thick Irish accent.

'And mine is Miss Sunshine,' she replied, holding her hand out to his.

Jay Bannerman didn't even hide the groan that came out his mouth as he shook her hand. 'This is going to be a disaster, isn't it?'

For a second – at least in Skye's head – things froze. She was captured by the man sitting in front of her. Now she'd stopped focusing on everything else she realised just how handsome he was. Discounting the fact that every time he spoke that lilting accent sent a whole host of vibrations down her spine, even if he hadn't opened his mouth, and she'd seen him in a bar, this guy was hot.

Skye didn't mix business with pleasure. She'd never been interested in dating her colleagues.

But at least he was semi-smiling now, and she would take that.

Continue reading

MELTING DR GRUMPY'S FROZEN HEART
Scarlet Wilson

Available next month
millsandboon.co.uk

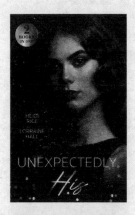
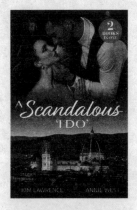
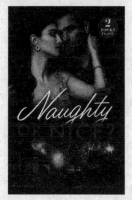
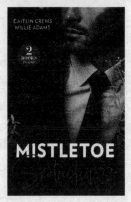

LET'S TALK
Romance

For exclusive extracts, competitions and special offers, find us online:

- **f** MillsandBoon
- **X** @MillsandBoon
- **⦿** @MillsandBoonUK
- **♪** @MillsandBoonUK

Get in touch on 01413 063 232

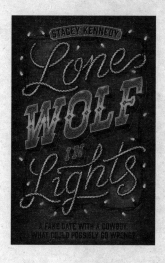
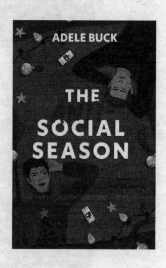

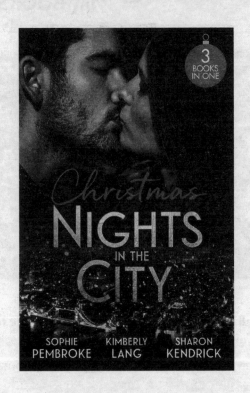

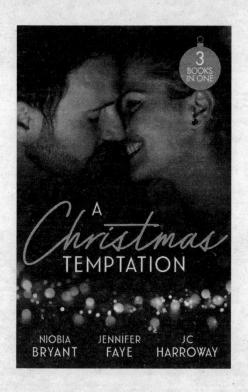

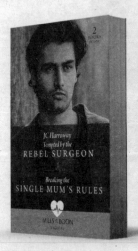 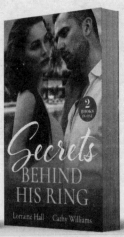 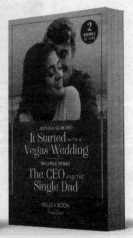